ARE WE READY?

CALIFORNIA/MILBANK BOOKS ON HEALTH AND THE PUBLIC

ARE WE READY?

PUBLIC HEALTH SINCE 9/11

David Rosner and Gerald Markowitz

UNIVERSITY OF CALIFORNIA PRESS
BERKELEY   LOS ANGELES   LONDON

MILBANK MEMORIAL FUND
NEW YORK

The Milbank Memorial Fund is an endowed operating foundation that engages in nonpartisan analysis, study, research, and communication on significant issues in health policy. In the Fund's own publications, in reports or books it publishes with other organizations, and in articles it commissions for publication by other organizations, the Fund endeavors to maintain the highest standards for accuracy and fairness. Statements by individual authors, however, do not necessarily reflect opinions or factual determinations of the Fund. For more information, visit www.milbank.org.

University of California Press, one of the most distinguished university presses in the United States, enriches lives around the world by advancing scholarship in the humanities, social sciences, and natural sciences. Its activities are supported by the UC Press Foundation and by philanthropic contributions from individuals and institutions. For more information, visit www.ucpress.edu.

University of California Press
Berkeley and Los Angeles, California

University of California Press, Ltd.
London, England

© 2006 by The Regents of the University of California

Library of Congress Cataloging-in-Publication Data

Rosner, David, 1947–
    Are we ready? : public health since 9/11 / David Rosner and Gerald Markowitz.
        p. ; cm. — (California/Milbank books on health and the public ; 15)
    Includes bibliographical references and index.
    ISBN-13: 978-0-520-24920-2 (cloth : alk. paper)
    ISBN-10: 0-520-24920-8 (cloth : alk. paper)
    ISBN-13: 978-0-520-25038-3 (pbk. : alk. paper)
    ISBN-10: 0-520-25038-9 (pbk. : alk. paper)
        1. Medical policy — United States. 2. Emergency medical services — United States. 3. Emergency management — United States. 4. September 11 Terrorist Attacks, 2001 — Health aspects — New York (State) — New York.
        [DNLM: 1. Public Policy — New York City. 2. Public Policy — United States. 3. September 11 Terrorist Attacks — New York City. 4. September 11 Terrorist Attacks — United States. 5. Bioterrorism — New York City. 6. Bioterrorism — United States. 7. Disaster Planning — New York City. 8. Disaster Planning — United States. 9. Government — New York City. 10. Government — United States. 11. Needs Assessment — New York City. 12. Needs Assessment — United States. WA 295 R822a 2006] I. Markowitz, Gerald E. II. Milbank Memorial Fund. III. Title. IV. Series.
    RA395.A3R66 2006
    362.18 — dc22   2006007396

Manufactured in the United States of America

15   14   13   12   11   10   09   08   07   06
10   9   8   7   6   5   4   3   2   1

CONTENTS

FOREWORD

The Milbank Memorial Fund is an endowed operating foundation that works to improve health by helping decision makers in the public and private sectors acquire and use the best available evidence to inform policy for health care and population health. The Fund has engaged in nonpartisan analysis and research on and communication about significant issues in health policy since its inception in 1905.

Are We Ready? Public Health since 9/11 is the fifteenth of the California/Milbank Books on Health and the Public. The publishing partnership between the Fund and the University of California Press seeks to encourage the synthesis and communication of findings from research that could contribute to more effective health policy.

David Rosner and Gerald Markowitz provide a history of governmental response to the effects on health of the terrorist attacks of September 11, 2001, and the subsequent anthrax cases. Their book is based on interviews with officials in New York City, many states, and the federal government and on written sources.

The authors document the dedication and insight of many senior officials of the legislative and executive branches of government. In the years since 9/11, these leaders have prepared for future disasters as tax revenues declined and the costs of health care and defense increased. As a result, the hurricanes of 2005 revealed both strengths and weaknesses of preparedness. Rosner and Markowitz address the response to the hurricanes in the preface, which was written while their book was in press.

The Fund published most of chapters 1 and 2 of this book as Milbank Reports in 2003 and 2004. The reports in this series result from the Fund's work with decision makers. The Fund invites decision makers who are interviewed for or quoted in a Milbank Report to review it in draft. Other decision makers and, as appropriate, researchers review each report for clarity and relevance. The Fund permits the authors of Milbank Reports to disagree with, but never to ignore, comments by reviewers. Because of the generally enthusiastic response of public officials to the first two reports and the draft of what would have been a third, the Fund and the Press invited Rosner and Markowitz to recast the reports and the manuscript as a book.

Daniel M. Fox
President

Samuel L. Milbank
Chairman

PREFACE

This book was completed before the tragedy that destroyed much of
New Orleans and the Gulf Coast in the late summer of 2005, when
thousands were left homeless and hundreds dead after Hurricane Katrina
struck. Like those who responded to the attacks of September 11, 2001,
those on the ground in the days after the hurricane inundated the region
performed heroically while working among the most dangerous conditions imaginable. Pulling people from attics, off roofs, out of polluted
water, and from the Superdome often demanded great courage on the
part of victim and rescuer alike.

The effort to provide food, shelter, services and ultimately homes to
thousands of people displaced by the disaster illustrated some of the most
wonderful qualities of Americans of all races, religions, and regions. The
experiences of San Antonio and other municipalities in Texas give us a
window into the extraordinary willingness of local communities to help
meet the needs of other Americans. According to State Senator Leticia
Van de Putte, who represents San Antonio, the state received somewhere
between a quarter and a half million evacuees from Louisiana alone. In
San Antonio fully 17,000 people were offered shelter by city agencies,
local churches, and Kelly USA, the former Kelly Air Force Base.

In part this was a very local response of people opening their hearts
after the tragedy of their neighbors in Louisiana, but in part it was also a
product of planning by local and state governments united by a formal
compact, the Emergency Management Assistance Compact (EMAC), set

up in 1995 to join Texas, Louisiana, Oklahoma, and Arkansas. Following 9/11, the states had added language to allow for reciprocal recognition of other states' health professionals "and other professionals as needed" during times of emergency. The practical impact has been enormous: teachers, social workers, engineers, nurses, doctors, and even cosmetologists who had been licensed in Louisiana were automatically certified to practice up to a year in Texas without having to go through the formal state licensing procedures. Similarly, those individuals who had received Medicaid in Louisiana were automatically provided care in Texas facilities. Job fairs, housing, a waiver of the usual deposit required for phone and electricity service, and monetary relief all followed. Many in the Texas shelters were given their first full medical exam, and some for the first time were diagnosed and treated for chronic conditions such as diabetes, heart disease, and asthma. In San Antonio professors from the local medical schools asked their medical and nursing students to help assess all evacuees.

State Senator Van de Putte, who was trained as a pharmacist, volunteered in the Kelly shelter and other shelters many evenings and was strongly affected by the stories of the people she encountered. People came to the shelters with rat bites received when the rodents, trying to escape the floods, sought to climb on people half-submerged in water. She met many who had been trapped in their houses, desperate for help; they told her, "Nobody came. Nobody cared. We couldn't get out." Van de Putte was deeply moved by the pictures drawn by children in the shelters. A common theme, she says, was "water, water, water everywhere. But not blues, no greens. The water was all black and gray and brown." The generosity of Texans speaks to what is best in Americans in all walks of life. The response in San Antonio and other localities was "This is what we need to do. We will find the funds to do it somehow. We are not going to wait for the feds to come in." But the response in Washington, she believes, was "How are we going to play this, how are we going to spin this?"[1]

In many troubling ways, the disaster in the Gulf brings home the lessons we should have learned from 9/11 but have not. The Federal Emergency Management Agency and its state equivalents had a proud history of successfully dealing with natural and other disasters. We need only recall the role that FEMA and local agencies played in bringing relief to the victims of the Oklahoma City bombing in 1995, or to those displaced by the floods that ravaged the Midwest in the mid-1990s, to understand how vital this agency had become since its founding in 1979.

When, in 2003, the Bush administration first proposed collapsing FEMA into the Department of Homeland Security, many worried that subsuming a disaster relief agency within a larger bureaucracy aimed at forestalling terrorist attacks might compromise its effectiveness. First, some were concerned that the focus on the extraordinary — that is, terrorist — event could distract professionals in the agency from the threats from nature that were far more likely to occur. Second, critics feared that the agency would lose the resources needed for maintaining the infrastructure of services essential to its everyday functions, pointing particularly to the looming budget deficits at the local and state levels. Moneys that might have gone to FEMA would be redirected to antiterrorist activities. Third, others predicted that the morale of those in FEMA would be undermined as budget cuts, a leadership vacuum, and the new focus on terrorism weakened the agency's integrity.

All these fears were borne out after FEMA became part of the Department of Homeland Security. In contrast to James Witt, FEMA's director during the Clinton administration, the new director and many of the top administrators appointed by the Bush administration were novices in the world of emergency relief. Budget cuts in each year since its incorporation into DHS, the loss of important programs, and a reduction of almost five hundred personnel crippled the agency charged with protecting us from unexpected events. As Jane Bullock, a longtime veteran in FEMA and its chief of staff in the 1990s, put it: "The federal system that was perfected in the '90s has been deconstructed. . . . FEMA has been marginalized. There is one focus [in the Department of Homeland Security] and the focus is on terrorism."[2] It is clear that although the hurricane would have caused tremendous damage to New Orleans and the entire Gulf Coast whatever the government did or didn't do, the response — or rather, the lack of response — by FEMA and DHS made a terrible situation far worse.

The events of September 2005 should cause us to be skeptical of any assurances by the federal government regarding our preparedness for natural or unnatural disasters. As one member of the 9/11 Commission put it following Katrina's devastation, "We've had our first test, and we've failed miserably."[3] Further, they should also make us think twice about the artificial distinctions between the natural and the unnatural that have often marked the decisions made since September 11, 2001. As the interviews that we conducted with officials from local, state, and federal agencies and that form the core of this book reveal, few with hands-on experience with disease and emergency preparedness believe that an adequate response to terrorism — whether biological, chemical, or radiological — is possible without a strong and vibrant infrastructure for providing everyday services as well. As smallpox, anthrax, and other possible bioterrorist hazards become the focus of the administration's interest in public health, we are in danger of neglecting the institutions that protect us from avian flu, SARS (severe acute respiratory syndrome), and other threats to the health of Americans. What public health and emergency preparedness experts have proclaimed for years is that the best way to prepare for bioterrorism or terrorism in general is to have a strong infrastructure capable of identifying threats, whether these result from nature or from conscious attack. The same labs, personnel, and institutions required to allay the impact of everyday diseases are needed for addressing the occasional anthrax outbreak or threat from smallpox. In short, just as our focus on terrorism may have compromised our response to Hurricane Katrina, so too the administration's focus on bioterrorism may have compromised the local public health infrastructure. For the public health community, the moral that has eluded those focused solely on terrorism has long been obvious: to address a possible bioterrorist attack it is essential to have services available that can respond to the ongoing danger posed by infections and health threats of all kinds.

ACKNOWLEDGMENTS

The terrorist attacks on September 11, 2001, shocked all Americans. In just a few moments our sense of safety shattered as four airplanes attacked the American mainland for the first time in history. These attacks and the concerns about the possibility of bioterrorism following the anthrax episode a month later, together with the mobilization to inoculate thousands of health care workers and others for smallpox, led to this book.

The events of 2001 and 2002 made it apparent that those working in agencies involved with a variety of population and public health issues were, for the first time in decades, central to our response to the threats facing the nation. Hence, we felt it imperative to document as fully as possible the experiences of public and population health workers, thereby developing a resource for policy makers and scholars in future years. This goal led to contact with the Robert Wood Johnson Foundation and an application for a grant to conduct oral histories with public health personnel in New York City who had been involved in the response to 9/11 and the anthrax attacks that occurred soon after. In January 2002, the Robert Wood Johnson Foundation provided David Rosner and Nancy VanDevanter with a Presidential Award to conduct thirty oral histories with first responders to the attacks and to process them and deposit them in the Oral History Collection at Columbia University. We are extremely grateful to James Knickman, vice president for research and evaluation at the Robert Wood Johnson Foundation, for his immediate and enthusiastic understanding of the importance of documenting the experiences of this community during this extremely stressful time. Further, we would like to thank Mary Marshall Clark, director of Columbia's Oral History Office, for her aid in processing these initial interviews. Nancy VanDevanter was, of course, a critical contributor in those early months, and we are grateful for her important role in conducting many of the interviews and providing initial contact with administrators in the New York City Department of Health.

As we were interviewing city workers about their immediate experiences with September 11, two simultaneous events spurred us to begin to expand our vision. First, Daniel Fox, president of the Milbank Memorial Fund, contacted us, asking if we would be interested in writing three reports for the Fund on the public health response to 9/11. The first report would build on our oral histories and other interviews that the Fund would support and would focus on the local New York City efforts to address the variety of problems for population health presented by the attacks. The second report would look at the reaction of the states, and the third report would focus on the Centers for Disease Control and Prevention and the federal response. Unlike the formal oral histories supported by the Robert Wood Johnson Foundation, these reports would be built around a much larger number of shorter interviews done with officials across the country.

Second, we received a Robert Wood Johnson Investigator Award to write a book tentatively titled "The Un-Natural History of Public Health," a volume that would reevaluate public health history in light of the events of September 11. In this project we hoped to reconceptualize disease and mortality patterns in American history as a reflection of the worlds we build and the social relationships that determine how we live and die. We are grateful to David Mechanic, director, and Lynn Rogut, deputy director, of RWJ's Investigator Awards in Health Policy Research. From the very beginning of our work they have been enthusiastic supporters of our efforts and we want to acknowledge our deep appreciation.

In our original Investigator Award proposal, 9/11, anthrax, and the smallpox campaign were to be the final chapters of a larger story and, as we continue to work on this project, they remain integrally connected to that broader account. But discussions with Daniel Fox and Kathleen Andersen at Milbank, as well as the discussions that took place about our work at the annual meetings of the Robert Wood Johnson scholars' retreat, led us to rethink our plan. It was clear that two books were emerging: the present volume and a reconceptualization of the history of disease in America. Without the help of the Milbank Memorial Fund and the Robert Wood Johnson Foundation, the scope of our thinking and our scholarly work would have remained much more limited.

This book would never have been possible without the extraordinary dedication of a band of graduate students at the Center for the History and Ethics of Public Health at Columbia's Mailman School of Public Health who have been essential in every aspect of the oral histories, interviews, data collection, and bibliographic research. Ben Fader, Rochelle Frounfelker, Marion Jones, Valeri Kiesig, Sheena Morrison, Elizabeth Robillotti, Molly Rosner, Zachary Rosner, Nicholas Turse, Sarah Vogel, and Megan Wolff were always helpful, insightful, and enthusiastic aides who generously gave of their time and energy at various points in this project. We are also grateful to a freelance copyeditor, Alice Falk, for careful, intelligent reading and suggestions as the manuscript neared completion.

Of course, the faculty and staff in our Center for the History and Ethics of Public Health, the Department of Sociomedical Sciences, the Mailman School of Public Health, Columbia's History Department, John Jay's Interdisciplinary Studies Program and History Department, and the CUNY Graduate Center's History Department were their usual funny, provocative, insightful, and wonderful selves. We must say that New York City provides an extraordinary working environment, filled with very special colleagues and friends. Priscilla Acuna, Andrea Balis, Ron Bayer, Betsy Blackmar, Michael Blitz, Steve Brier, Artie Brown, Josh Brown, Jim Cohen, James Colgrove, Pat Collins, Blanche Wiesen Cook, Andrew Davidson, Eli Faber, Amy Fairchild, Eric Foner, Josh Freeman, Mary Gibson, Betsy Gitter, Don Goodman, Carol Groneman, Richard Haw, Alice Kessler-Harris, Sondra Leftoff, Barron Lerner, MaryAnn McClure, David Nasaw, Nitanya Nedd, Gerald Oppenheimer, Richard Parker, Ed Paulino, Irwin Redlener, Allan Rosenfield, Shirley Sarna, Kofi Scott, Dennis Sherman, Abby Stein, Fritz Umbach, Darryl Westcott-Marshall, Basil Wilson, and Michael Yudell all helped us with their insights and goodwill as well as constant support.

Of course, this book depends heavily on the extraordinary group of people in the various city, state, and federal agencies whose interviews and/or reviews form its intellectual content. We can't thank them enough for their willingness to speak honestly about their experiences during what was clearly one of the most trying periods of their professional lives: Barbara Aaron, Mimi Abramovitz, John O. Agwunobi, Tom Allen,

Brian W. Amy, J. Nick Baird, Edward L. Baker, Georges Benjamin, Susan Blank, Michael Caldwell, Jan K. Carney, Ronald Cates, Harriette Chandler, John Chapin, J. Jarrett Clinton, Jack Colley, Angela Coron, Tim Daly, George DiFerdinando Jr., Robert B. Eadie, Catherine Eden, David Engelthaler, Ann Marie Fraschilla, Thomas E. Gecewicz, Andrew Goodman, Richard Gottfried, Lee Greenfield, Norma Gyle, George Hardy, Anne Harnish, Joseph Henderson, Doug Hensel, John Howard, James Hughes, Joseph Hunt, C. Earl Hunter, Joseph P. Iser, Richard Jackson, Igal Jellinek, Lisa Kaplowitz, Dan Kass, David Klasfeld, Jeffrey Koplan, Mary Kramer, Rachel Kramer, Jack Krauskopf, Keith Kutler, Marci Layton, Rice Leach, Alvin Lee, Stephen Levin, Scott Lillibridge, John R. Lumpkin, Ekaterina Malievskaia, Steven Markowitz, Sabrina Jaar Marzouka, Gene Matthews, Kelly McKinney, Patrick Meehan, A. Richard Melton, Dora Anne Mills, Scott Milstein, Carol M. Moehrle, Benjamin Mojica, Patricia T. Montoya, Stephen Morse, Tony Moulton, Sandra Mullin, Jerrold Nadler, Gail Nayowith, Melvin Neufeld, Patricia A. Nolan, Stephen Ostroff, Dennis Perrotta, Sheila Peterson, Richard A. Raymond, Peggy Reeves, Steven Rubin, Charlene Rydell, J. Thomas Schedler, Richard H. Schultz, Samuel Sebiyam, Mary C. Selecky, Donna Shelley, Steve Siegfried, Marvin A. Singleton, Arvy Smith, Kathy W. Stein, Robert B. Stroube, Ezra Susser, Ed Thompson, Kathleen E. Toomey, Leticia Van de Putte, Doris Varlese, Charlie Vitchers, Brenda Vossler, Susan Waltman, Janice L. Weinstein, Isaac Weisfuse, Lucindy Williams, and Robert S. Zimmerman Jr.

Finally, we want to acknowledge the friendship and support of Dean Allan Rosenfield. He has been a colleague in the truest sense of the word.

INTRODUCTION

Remembering the Moment

How can we understand the emotionally charged events surrounding September 11, 2001? How can we begin to comprehend the impact on our psyches, our institutions, and our people of the World Trade Center collapse, the attack on the Pentagon, and the crash of a jetliner in the fields of Pennsylvania? To what extent have these events permanently altered the political, cultural, and organizational life of the country? To what extent is the nation better prepared to withstand another potentially devastating attack? To what extent are we better prepared to deal with possible chemical, biological, or radiological attacks? Half a decade after the events, we can begin both to evaluate the impact of 9/11 on the nation's public health infrastructure and responses and to analyze the long-lasting, perhaps permanent, changes that have reshaped our public health system.

How best can we capture the immediacy of the moments when the planes hit? Perhaps most poignant are the memories of one official who, ironically, was then about as far removed from New York City as possible. Richard Jackson, at the time the director of the Centers for Disease Control and Prevention's National Center for Environmental Health, recalls that he had gone hiking as part of his annual vacation.

> On September 7 I went off to do my annual hike with my old med school roommates. . . . We were going to hike the Wind River wilderness in Montana. We started out in Green River lakes on about the 7th or 8th of September, and hiked up to about 11,000 feet, through the snow. . . . I'd left

my pager and cell phone, because I figured, "Even if there's a death in my family, I don't want to know about it. I just need to go and be alone, just chill out." I remember lying on a rock over an alpine meadow, and looking up at the sky — perfectly blue sky, and thinking, "God, I haven't seen the sky without a jet contrail in it for years. This is really remote."[1]

He had no idea that terrorist attacks had taken place until he was on his way out and "a backpacker coming in . . . told me that the World Trade Center had fallen down. I had family here in New York, including a couple of sisters. Obviously, I was very concerned about extended family. When I finally got out and was able to get to a pay phone that worked, my wife was frantic. I didn't appreciate until I got home just how psychologically traumatized even someone . . . living in Atlanta was, watching these images on TV and then just how stressful it had been."

While Jackson was enjoying his vacation, back in Atlanta at the CDC months of preparation were being put to the test. He says, "By five minutes after the first plane hit, they had already begun to mobilize. . . . People obviously didn't realize that this was a terrorist event for another twenty minutes or so, and when that began to dawn on people, the CDC headquarters were closed, and [soon] the CDC executive staff were moved out of the Clifton Road facility, and over to my center, which is about eight, ten miles away from the headquarters facility on a secure ex-naval air station." This emergency operations center was equipped "with TV screens and various clocks and very good and secure communications and the rest. . . . Barbed wires surround our laboratories and everything else." After 9/11, points out Jeffrey Koplan, then the director of the Centers for Disease Control and Prevention, "for the first time in history the people at the CDC in Atlanta themselves felt vulnerable. . . . We had a walled fortress for an entrance and armed police patrolling the halls whereas prior to September 11 the police were unarmed."[2] Jackson later learned that "on the afternoon of the 11th, Jeff Koplan and the CDC leadership were there in my offices, looking out at the Peachtree DeKalb Airport. . . . It's where all the corporate jets go in and out of, and we had a contract for the National Pharmaceutical Stockpile, to have a jet available if we needed it."

On September 11, 2001, the federal government activated the National Disaster Medical System and, over the course of the next two days, sent five teams of doctors, nurses, and emergency medical technicians to New York and four teams to the Pentagon; placed thirty-five CDC epidemiologists in hospitals in New York City; sent push packages containing 50 tons of medical supplies to New York; and, within four hours of the attack, used the CDC's Health Alert Network, a national online system for improving communication, to transmit health alerts and messages to public health officials.[3] Jackson recalls, "Every plane within the United States, with the exception of Air Force One and the military aircraft, was on the ground." In fact, "the only civilian plane to take off in the entire United States was the CDC-rented corporate jet, with F-16 escorts flying up . . . into LaGuardia. . . . It was very emotional. The senior staff said there were tears in their eyes, watching this plane take off." As he explains, "No one flies string lines directly into LaGuardia. You circle around. This plane went right over the World Trade Center. We have pictures our own staff took, looking down on the Trade Center. . . . Seeing the World Trade Center [site] — everyone was . . . stunned." After they landed, "they were dispersed to provide assistance to the New York City Health Department, to set up a response center at Pier 92, and to put staff in the hospitals to track who was coming in."

This book analyzes the impact of 9/11, the anthrax attacks that followed, and smallpox preparedness on the nation's public health infrastructure. Drawing on interviews with local, state, and federal officials, we have sought to explore the immediate reactions to these events by examining the recollections of people deeply involved in them. Each chapter concentrates on one level of government, including its interactions with the other levels. The first looks at the experiences of local New York officials who were the first responders as events unfolded and as state and national authorities arrived. The second chapter turns to the various states and the changes in their federal funding for numerous public and population health activities. The final chapter focuses on the federal response to 9/11 and the anthrax mailings, using oral histories of CDC and other federal officials. Together, they show officials at all levels of government reacting to 9/11 with extraordinary commitment and effort. What emerges is a picture of dedicated public servants who were, like the rest of us, overcome by the emotions of the moment yet whose response managed to considerably reduce public anxiety and the public health threat. Despite significant problems in formulating appropriate public health policies to prepare for bioterrorism, emergency responses, disease surveillance, inoculation, and laboratory testing, these city, state, and federal public health officials acted out of deep concern for the overall health of citizens all over the country.

Are We Ready? is a contemporary history of a critical period of time. The purpose of contemporary history is to tell the story as people experienced it, using a wide variety of primary sources — published and unpublished reports, oral interviews with key participants, government documents, popular media, and so on. Contemporary history is generally the first attempt to place its subject in a longer and broader historical context. Hence, it offers no specific recommendations to address the issues it raises. Rather, as all history tries to do, it seeks to provide perspective on contemporary issues that may or may not be incorporated into policy decisions. As historians, we hope to provide the reader with the lessons learned and insights gleaned by the participants themselves.

Because the interviews on which this book is based were conducted over the course of the four years since the attacks, they reflect the changing political, social, and economic environments of the country that obviously frame the interviewees' recollections and analyses. The first chapter details the experiences of officials and actors in the public health, social services, political, and educational communities in the immediate aftermath, when they were reacting within a highly charged and emotionally wrenching atmosphere. The candor with which these officials reported their experiences and anxieties is, therefore, all the more affecting. For the second chapter, we interviewed state officials who saw growing federal attention to the problems they faced and who initially hoped that the infusions of federal money and activity would bring long-term benefits to the public and population health infrastructure. But even within two years of the attacks, they could already see that state and federal budget constraints would curtail the promised improvements. By the time the third chapter was researched, three years after the attacks, federal officials were able to reflect on the accomplishments and the shortfalls of the efforts to improve the nation's public and population health.

This book comes at a time when we have largely been distracted from paying attention to the nation's security and especially to its preparations for bioterrorist, chemical, and nuclear terrorism by the pressing demands of the Iraq conflict and fiscal uncertainties at the local, state, and federal levels. Even after facing emergencies such as SARS (severe acute respiratory syndrome), monkeypox, and the shortage of influenza vaccine, we apparently — despite the very real improvements in many aspects of bioterrorism preparedness — have lost our sense of urgency in addressing the weaknesses of the public health infrastructure and the national need for its systematic reform. While most still remember where they were "when the planes hit," the shock of that terrorist attack has faded. As Gene Matthews, then legal advisor to the CDC and now director of the Institute of Public Health Law at Georgia State University, notes, "What happens is that first we are in a green zone of normal times (pre-9/11), then we get into a red zone where the culture changes after an epidemic or a bioterrorism emergency. Then we enter a gray zone where change takes place — for example, the Department of Homeland Security, bioterrorism grants, and so on. Then we go back to the green zone when we can't remember what it was like during a crisis."[4]

September 11 and anthrax, the threat of smallpox, and the continuing AIDS epidemic, as well as the more recent outbreaks of SARS and monkeypox and the threat of an avian flu pandemic, compelled general government — elected officials and their staffs — to pay more sustained attention and award resources to public health agencies and population health more broadly than it had done in decades. Here we distinguish between public health and population health services. By *public health* we mean those services aimed at preventing epidemics and the spread of disease; promoting chronic disease control and encouraging healthy behavior; preventing and responding to disasters; administering public health departments; and licensing and maintaining facilities, vital records, and laboratories. In *population health* we include those services normally rendered by public health departments as well as those that provide access to personal health services of high quality; ensure financial security for parents of young children and retirees; protect against harm as a result of poor water quality, air pollution, toxic soil, and contaminated food; control risks from tobacco and other addictive substances; reduce injuries and risk of illness in workplaces, homes, and public spaces; and protect the independence of persons who are frail or have disabilities.[5]

This shifting terrain reminds us of the importance of political and economic realities in shaping our perceptions of what public and population health are and are not. As James Hughes, director of the CDC's National Center for Infectious Diseases, astutely observes, "You of course know Bill Foege [a former director of the CDC], who said that public health is where politics and science come together. We are at that interface."[6]

ONE

SEPTEMBER 11 AND THE SHIFTING PRIORITIES OF PUBLIC AND POPULATION HEALTH IN NEW YORK CITY

September 11, 2001, affected virtually all aspects of American life, from foreign policy and domestic security to philanthropy, social services, and health policy. Social welfare, public health, health care, and environmental issues, generally seen as separate spheres, are now increasingly understood as interrelated components essential to the mental and social well-being and emergency preparedness of a traumatized nation and city, and the opportunities to integrate these concerns are immense. The experience of 9/11 has highlighted the interrelationships between biological, sanitary, medical, social, and economic factors that together affect the well-being of populations. Perhaps more directly than any other recent event, analysts point out, September 11 has illustrated that a population's health "encompasses a broader array of determinants of health than the field of public health has previously addressed," making all the more critical the "emerging theory and practice of population health" — one that incorporates "the traditional concerns of public health" with "such issues as the effects on health status of . . . relative income and social status, racial and gender disparities, and educational achievement."[1]

This chapter is organized both chronologically and thematically. We begin by reviewing the immediate response of New York City's Department of Health to the attack on the World Trade Center and the subsequent anthrax episode. We then analyze the difficulty of establishing responsible policies to aid the city's and nation's return to normalcy in the face of enormous scientific uncertainty about the potential health hazards of dust, debris, and toxic materials in the neighborhoods and schools near the World Trade Center site. Finally, we address the special immediate threats that the disaster posed to the population's health. Of particular importance were the social service and mental health sectors, largely organized through voluntary agencies: we discuss the immediate and longer-term responses of these agencies and the problems they encountered as they adjusted to long-term population health needs. Thus we begin with the narrowest conceptions of health as defined by the activities of the New York Department of Health and broaden our study to include the agencies and issues that affect population health policy.

The immediate response to the attack on the World Trade Center showed the surprising strength of New York City's existing public health and social welfare infrastructure, but the attack also revealed important weaknesses that will have to be addressed in the future. Though the decentralized system of social and public health services was in some respects an advantage in responding to unpredictable and varied disasters, the need for a greater degree of centralization of services and control was nevertheless apparent. At times the political and public health leadership effectively communicated what was known and not known about the dangers to residents' health and welfare, while at other times political leaders with differing agendas propagated a confusing array of messages, leading to uncertainty and distrust among the broader public.

The history we relate in the following pages must be understood as being deeply imbedded in ongoing political and social struggles around political power, race, neighborhood redevelopment, immigration, and the responsibilities of New York City's largely voluntary social service system. Despite the ubiquity of the image of "a nation united" in the weeks after 9/11, in reality the depiction of the events, almost from the first minutes after the attack, was shaped by continuing social divisions between rich and poor, between black, Hispanic, and white, and even between Republicans and Democrats. For example, Joseph Bruno, the New York State Senate majority leader, was quick to compare the responses to 9/11 in the two communities most directly affected: New York and Washington. In New York, Bruno argued, an efficient and well-ordered emergency response system mobilized a vast array of resources that, under the leadership of Governor George Pataki and Mayor Rudolph Giuliani, both Republicans, calmed the public and answered the immediate needs of a traumatized community. As Bruno put it, "The leadership they provided moments after the disaster came after years of putting together an excellent response plan." But in

Washington, D.C., Bruno maintained, the lack of effective local political leadership and absence of an emergency plan led to a confused, disjointed set of decisions that fell short in calming the public or providing needed services. He declared, "Local leaders [can] look to Washington, D.C., and New York City for dramatic examples of one city that wasn't prepared to respond to terrorist attacks and another that was."[2] Certainly, Bruno gave major credit for the success of New York's response effort to the Republican leadership of the city and state, contrasting it with the Democratic local leadership in Washington, D.C., and effectively ignoring the unique control exercised over local government in Washington by Congress (indeed, at the time the city's finances were being overseen by a presidentially appointed control board); moreover, he failed to mention that the attack was in Northern Virginia, while Washington itself was untouched.

Here we turn a skeptical eye on the underlying politics that have driven the city's reaction to September 11. We take for granted that the response of the city's political leadership was shaped by existing social tensions, as well as a physical, governmental, and nonprofit infrastructure that was put in place throughout the twentieth century — especially during the administration of Fiorello La Guardia (1934–45) and in the decades after World War II, when New York experimented with a wide range of public health and social welfare programs.[3] In contrast to Bruno's portrayal, which personalizes New Yorkers' "successful" response, we argue that implicit national priorities distorted how health and welfare policies were implemented in the period following the attacks. How effectively the city and state responded to the emergency rested only in part on their political leadership, the planning done by the State Emergency Management Office (SEMO), or even the Federal Emergency Management Agency (FEMA), although all played a role.

THE EMERGENCY RESPONSE IN THE HOURS AFTER THE ATTACK

Although the city initially took the lead in the emergency response, certain state and federal agencies were involved in coordinating aid and resources that flowed in from elsewhere in the state and across the nation. Since 1996, New York State has had in place an emergency management office charged with responding to the natural disasters that may cripple different areas of the state. Ice storms in the Adirondacks, hurricanes on Long Island, droughts in the apple-growing districts in the center of the state, and other emergencies caused by weather have been its primary focus since the mid-1990s. In 2000, the anticipated computer meltdown that never occurred, "the Y2K bug," broadened the mandate of the office beyond natural disasters. But though the World Trade Center (WTC) had been targeted by terrorists and seriously damaged in a 1993 bombing, the office was unprepared for the dimensions of the attack that occurred on September 11, 2001. Within moments, a social as well as physical disaster overwhelmed the agencies that were normally expected to deal with disaster relief.

The State Emergency Management Office helped coordinate the immediate response. SEMO called on thirty-one emergency experts from eighteen states associated with the Emergency Management Assistance Compact (EMAC) — a mutual aid agreement among states that was initially intended to address natural disasters such as hurricanes, wildfires, and toxic waste spills as well as acts of terrorism — to help manage logistics and donations. (New York was not formally part of EMAC before September 11 but joined it through state legislative action in the days after the attack.)[4] Five other states also sent specialists in disaster relief. Through SEMO, 5,000 National Guard troops, 500 state troopers and K-9 units, 100 Bureau of Criminal Investigation personnel, and 2,500 crisis counselors were dispatched to the city. The State Department of Health provided 400 workers to the New York City Department of Health to expedite the issuance of death certificates for families of victims, to monitor air quality, and to coordinate volunteer personnel. In addition, the New York State Insurance Department, Empire State Development Corporation, Department of Transportation, and Department of Labor all provided a host of services.

The Federal Emergency Response

For some in the New York City Department of Health, the real "white knights" — to use the words of Kelly McKinney, the department's associate commissioner of regulatory and environmental health services — were the federal emergency response experts who appeared in the hours following the attack. Local health officials were appreciative of experts like Ron Burger, senior emergency response coordinator with the Centers for Disease Control and Prevention (CDC), who had extensive experience with all sorts of natural disasters and who seemed unfazed by the events. Burger was among a small group of experts from the CDC and the Department of Health and Human Services that arrived in New York City on the afternoon of September 11. McKinney describes him as "sort of geeky in a lovable way. . . . He's got his CDC polo shirt with the pen around the neck and the emergency response I.D. card and the boots and stuff. . . . He's done this so many times. He probably sleeps in that." At meetings of the mayor's emergency response team, McKinney said, rather than telling everyone what to do Burger would sit there and listen: "He's a fly on the wall, and every once in a while he'd say something . . . and he'll sort of nudge you a little bit [and soon] he'll say something and then the lightbulb would go on. All of a sudden, you'd say, 'Oh, I see.'"[5]

The lines of authority were frequently confused and unclear as federal, state, and local officials tried to give (or had to take) orders from their counterparts at different levels of government. McKinney remembers that at one meeting, representatives from the Coast Guard and the Environmental Protection Agency (EPA) both were giving guidance to city officials. "They knew this stuff had to be done. . . . They had to get the city to request it," McKinney recalls. "They were looking for someone to request it. Anybody that was walking by, they grabbed them: 'Can you just request . . . this. Can you request?' People would be like, 'Get away from me.'" These early moments of chaos were overcome, but small and large conflicts over who had authority at any given moment would create ongoing problems in the weeks and months ahead.

The Immediate Hospital Response

In the minutes and hours following the attack on the World Trade Center, an astounding array of emergency vehicles — from fire trucks and police vans to ambulances from hospitals all over the city — gathered along the West Side Highway above Canal Street awaiting word about when to drive downtown to the disaster site to provide relief and pick up the injured. Lining the highway for blocks were ambulances from virtually every hospital in Manhattan: Mt. Sinai, NYU Downtown Hospital, New York Presbyterian, Bellevue, and others. The ambulances sat and sat as it became apparent that few of them were needed for the anticipated massive casualties: the terrorist attack had left many victims but few survivors.

Like their ambulance services, the hospitals throughout the New York region had readied themselves for an onslaught of what they imagined would be thousands of patients who had survived the attack. They emptied their wards and rooms of all but the most seriously ill and mobilized their staffs to await the ambulances they expected would soon arrive at emergency room entrances. Hours went by as doctors, nurses, orderlies, and technicians streamed to the institutions. Yet, like the ambulance services, they found that they were not needed. In the following days, administrators complained that their institutions had absorbed enormous costs as the emptied beds and canceled services had deprived them of revenue. Who, they asked, should bear the costs of an emergency mobilization spurred by a sense of patriotism and civic duty? In the end, the hospitals themselves bore the loss.

The city's hospitals had, through the Greater New York Hospital Association, made an enormous effort in the late 1990s to make sure they were prepared for the potential chaos that might ensue from a citywide crash of computers as a result of the Y2K bug. Susan Waltman and Doris Varlese, the association's general counsel and assistant general counsel, respectively, agreed that "the extensive preparation and drilling done for Y2K were vital to the preparedness of New York area hospitals on 9/11."[6] "Though at the time some criticized the amount of money and attention spent to deal with a Y2K disaster that never materialized, 9/11 proved that the efforts were not wasted," regardless of the relatively small number of actual casualties, points out Waltman.[7] Varlese recalls that she was with the mayor at "ground zero" shortly after the first plane hit and was at the fire station where the emergency headquarters was set up. "Though they did not have the technology and equipment that would have been available to them in the regular emergency headquarters," she notes, "things functioned effectively and efficiently because everyone had been so well trained."

The episode reveals the enormous resources available in New York and demonstrates that the institutions themselves were able to implement emergency protocols quickly and efficiently, despite all the initial chaos and the lack of clarity as to the disaster's true extent or nature. Yet even though the state had a disaster preparedness plan on the books, observes Richard Gottfried, New York State Assembly member from Manhattan and chair of the Assembly Committee on Health, the Greater New York Hospital Association, among many others, testified at an Assembly Health Committee hearing that it "had no interaction with the disaster preparedness council that was supposed to implement the plan." Indeed, the disaster plan had not been updated since the early 1990s and for all practical purposes "did not function" during the crisis.

The Role of Voluntary Agencies

The day-to-day efforts to meet the needs of the city fell to voluntary agencies — that is, organizations that run on a nonprofit basis, with tax-exempt status from the state — and departments of the city government, and many were struck by the order and coordination that marked those early days and weeks. Richard Jackson, then director of the CDC's National Center for Environmental Health, reflects: "Never in my whole career had I ever experienced a sense of superb management and seamless coordination around a series of important issues. It could not have functioned more effectively. . . . I hate to say this, but New York was absolutely the best place in the country for this to happen, only because the networks of personnel, knowing who your peers were, knowing how the system would work, confidence in them, seamless communications whether electronic or otherwise, really had been pretty much set up."[8]

THE NEW YORK CITY DEPARTMENT OF HEALTH

In the hours after the planes hit, the department's various officials and staff were drawn into some of the most basic tasks of caring for people in crisis. Because it was located just a few blocks away from the World Trade Center, and because its staff was arriving at work at the very moment of the attack, the Department of Health was literally well positioned to mobilize an early response effort.

Providing Immediate Help

In the hours after the attack, Department of Health personnel provided emergency services to injured people who were streaming uptown from ground zero. Susan Blank, assistant commissioner of the department's Sexually Transmitted Disease Control Program, remembers people coming into 125 Worth Street "truly covered in ash. Before, some people had like, yes, ash, but these people were caked in ash, their nostrils really covered in ash. People were singed, mucous membranes, people who were freaked. There were firefighters who came in here, there were police officers who came in here, there were citizens who came in here." Although the Department of Health headquarters on Worth Street, near City Hall, "was not ever envisioned as a clinic site,"[9] and was not equipped to deliver any direct services, the staff rose to the occasion and converted the lobby of the building into a triage center where people were treated for dust inhalation and eye irritation as well as scrapes, heart palpitations, and broken bones.

Staff was called in from a variety of clinics around the city to serve as an emergency medical corps. Lucindy Williams, the clinic manager for

STD clinics in Fort Greene and Williamsburg in Brooklyn and on Staten Island, recalls that she and other physicians from her clinic in Fort Greene immediately left Brooklyn with "a policeman and a police car escort[ing] us across the bridge to Manhattan."[10] "We were here," remembers Isaac Weisfuse, the Department of Health's deputy commissioner for disease control, "and in the meantime they started bringing in casualties. That's something we actually never really prepared ourselves to deal with, because at the Health Department we have STD clinics and tuberculosis clinics, but we're not really a casualty" center. "Thankfully, they didn't bring anybody with more than broken bones."[11] In fact, there is no reason why the Department of Health *should* have been prepared to deal with casualties, since it is the role of the city's Emergency Medical Services and trauma systems to provide such services.

But while the department tried to adjust to the immediate demands placed on it for medical care, its major focus was, in fact, on very traditional public health issues. Benjamin Mojica, then deputy commissioner of health and director of the division of health, recalls coming out of the subway, on his way to jury duty, to see people staring at the North Tower, which had just been hit by the first plane. He quickly altered his plan for the day and went to his office, just across the street in the Foley Square complex of government buildings. He called in his emergency response team and organized a meeting in the conference room on the third floor at 125 Worth Street.[12] The meeting mobilized almost every unit of the department. Their plans included monitoring air quality, coordinating with other agencies to see to the safety of search and rescue workers, tracking illness and injuries at New York City hospitals, monitoring water quality around ground zero, inspecting food establishments below Canal Street, overseeing the distribution of food for rescue workers, and surveying the impact of the blast on rodent activity.

Traditional Public Health Services

There were two hundred restaurants and other food outlets in the immediate area around the WTC, as Mojica points out, "with spoiling food. In addition to the stench . . . there's going to be a potential for rodents to invade the area and help themselves to this big supply of food that was left behind." Working with other city agencies to mobilize inspectors, exterminators, and cleanup crews to "abate conditions conducive to rodent harborage," the Department of Health set about to enter restaurants that had been abandoned by owners, where decaying food was creating a tremendous insect and rodent problem. Mojica notes that he didn't "know how many tons of food we threw out, . . . but it took us almost three weeks to" clear the restaurants, food shops, and supermarkets of huge quantities of rotting matter.

Because restaurant inspectors were called downtown in the emergency, there were no restaurant inspections or rodent control activities north of Canal Street for nearly a month. No births were registered for about two weeks in New York City. And because the department was so focused on the possibility of bioterrorism, its sole investigatory activity was to monitor infectious diseases that appeared in hospitals. According to Mojica, no "regular, routine" surveillance of non-terrorist-related diseases or conditions occurred.

In addition, the Department of Health established systems to monitor emergency departments to assess acute injuries, oversaw hospital staffing and equipment needs, watched for unusual disease patterns that could indicate a bioterrorist event, issued medical advisories to the public and medical community, and "facilitated development and coordination of environmental sampling."[13] In the hours immediately following the attack, the department began to conduct "swipings" in the area around the site to test for bioterrorism and chemical agents.

Contrary to much of the rhetoric about the impact of 9/11 on redirecting the priorities of public health, the experience in fact highlighted how essential to dealing with the emergency were traditional public health functions: record keeping, disease monitoring, pest control, water safety, sewerage treatment, and disposal and sanitation.

Environmental Health at Ground Zero

The Department of Health took charge of providing respiratory equipment to the workers who began to sift through the rubble in the days immediately following the attack. It thus had the responsibility of fitting masks and respirators to every person on every shift. Andrew Goodman, the department's associate commissioner of community health works, recalls the "enormous effort by a team of people at the Health Department to organize the procurement and then the distribution of 20,000 to 30,000 respirators." He adds, "We were down at ground zero trying to figure out respirators, and we would have masks from one company and filters from another and it took actually a few days before we had a system set up where we could get masks out to everybody . . . probably thousands of firefighters, police, and other rescue workers."[14]

Isaac Weisfuse recalls that he "couldn't believe how many masks and other things we were getting in. . . . It didn't dawn on me until a day or two later that there were thousands of new people showing up every day, who weren't fit tested . . . and I think threw [the masks] away at the end of the day, thinking they didn't have to keep them . . . but we went through a ton of masks."

Susan Blank remembers the difficulties of deciding what materials could be used at the disaster site. Although donations were pouring in, each item of equipment — even bottled water, for example — had to be evaluated as to its source and safety. "There were discussions about, can we accept donated supplies? Maybe they're laced with some agent of bioterrorism. . . . So we can't accept these types of donations; we have to turn them back. Yeah, but the workers are out there working but they're unprotected. If you look at the early news pictures, they weren't wearing masks." Two other major concerns in the first days following the attack, points out Benjamin Mojica, were how to get potable water to the disaster site and the need to address the danger from "potential cross-contamination of the water from sewage and other effluents" following the dramatic drop in water pressure caused by the large number of hoses and fire hydrants the fire department had opened.

Goodman argues that "the infrastructure [wa]s not as strong as it could be, certainly in terms of our capability to do surveillance at the level that we truly like and really also utilizing technology that is currently available." Some traced the problem to long-term trends in public health, as attention to chronic disease problems had grown and concern about epidemic diseases had declined over the course of the past half century. Some Department of Health officials complained that the increasing funds flowing into the hospital system and the growing prestige of medicine and medical technology (as antibiotics, polio vaccine, and transplantation, among many other biomedical techniques, were developed) had drained the public health field of resources and prestige. New York's fiscal crisis of the 1970s led to a shrinkage of the department's budget in real dollars, creating a major crisis that forced it to close clinics, limit its number of inspectors, reduce infectious disease surveillance, and reduce its central office workforce.

But the advent of the AIDS epidemic in the 1980s and 1990s, the shorter-term crisis caused by a spike in tuberculosis in the late 1980s, and the special attention to West Nile virus in recent years had helped draw the city's attention to the vital role played by the Department of Health and had underscored the importance of supporting the department's traditional functions.[15] Still, at the time of the attack, though major improvements had occurred, some parts of the department remained weak; specifically, its laboratories, once seen as the jewels in its crown, had fallen on hard times.[16]

The Department of Health not only had to react to the emergency itself but also had to be "anticipatory" of coming problems associated with the relationship between ongoing public health needs and the cleanup activities. Weisfuse recalls that "it was West Nile season, and there were all these hoses and water." He and other department personnel worried, "Are all the firemen going to get West Nile?" With literally millions of gallons of water being poured onto the smoldering fires that continued to burn for months after the attack, the site itself became a perfect breeding ground. Hence, the department began to identify standing pools of water and to lace them with insecticides to ward off what might have been a massive problem.

The Anthrax Episode

While the attack on the World Trade Center highlighted the Department of Health as essential and exposed the limitations in its ability to fulfill its enormous mandate, the anthrax episode further tested its ability to respond to the city's needs. On September 25, an assistant to Tom Brokaw, the NBC news anchor, opened a letter filled with white powder and handled a second letter that contained some kind of sandy substance, and her supervisors called the FBI. Three days later the employee developed symptoms — a "strange sore on her chest" — and her doctor, evidently suspecting anthrax, prescribed the antibiotic Cipro. The NBC employee also visited a dermatologist, and one of her physicians contacted the New York City Department of Health to test the powder; it was found to be negative for anthrax. But the biopsy of the sore was sent to the CDC, which did identify anthrax. At first the city and federal agencies failed to communicate, and the *New York Times* reported that "coordinating the efforts of the various law enforcements and public health officials [proved] tricky."[17] But the experience they had gained from running STD and TB clinics enabled city officials, though stretched to their limits, to quickly organize a method for distributing Cipro and providing other services necessary to identify victims and find sources of infection.[18]

The strengths and weaknesses revealed in the city's public health infrastructure by the mailing of anthrax to NBC became manifest on a national scale when postal workers were discovered to have been exposed to the deadly substance. Neither the CDC nor the Defense Department nor any other agencies could cope with the escalating demands to test suspicious powders or secure sites thought to be contaminated. In particular, the city's own laboratory was overwhelmed by the huge number of samples flooding it and was made inoperable by the lack of trained staff. Although only four cases of anthrax were identified, New York City could not keep up with the thousands of tests it needed to run on matter from humans and from the environment; and because the staff as well as the police and others who brought in samples lacked training or experience, proper handling of the material was difficult and sometimes impossible.[19] Indeed, at one point the department's laboratories at East 26th Street were themselves contaminated by anthrax; they became functional again only after the army brought in its own mobile emergency laboratory, which was set up in the lobby. Though members of the laboratory staff were working twenty-four hours a day and doing an extraordinary job, they became the scapegoats because they were not returning specimens quickly enough. "We were really overwhelmed by the response from the community," Ben Mojica recalls, "and the number of specimens we received in the laboratory. There were thousands of them."

A semblance of order returned to the labs after the Defense Department intervened and established a mobile laboratory, following requests from the mayor to Secretary of Defense Donald Rumsfeld. But new tensions emerged, as officials feared the possible "militarization" of public health activities. The anthrax episode, an emergency requiring an immediate response to the threat of bioterrorism, created an uneasy alliance between military and public health cultures. Public health generally has been a methodical, sometimes slow, science of investigation, and new demands, especially for speed, were being made on it.

Further, the experience with the postal workers in the midtown Manhattan mail handling facility (and in the Brentwood facility in Washington, D.C.) exposed the flaws in a decentralized public health system. There were no clear national guidelines for who should be tested for anthrax, who should be given Cipro as a preventive measure, what should be done after anthrax spores were identified in a facility. As a reporter noted, "The individual incidents where anthrax has actually been found have been handled differently by health and law enforcement officials on each scene, leading to confusion and anger in some areas."[20]

Though the infrastructure itself was at times immobilized by the demands placed on it, the city's population reacted with remarkable calm to the events that were being reported daily over local and national television and other news media. In some measure this can be attributed to Mayor Rudy Giuliani's handling of the anthrax episode. The mayor held daily press conferences that provided relatively full and accurate information about the scope of the problem, giving a detailed account of what was being done to deal with the threat; he avoided speculation while offering a degree of reassurance to a nervous city. In essence, he "appealed to people's most rational selves" and counted on the public to reach reasonable conclusions about the real scope of the threat and on public officials to act responsibly and appropriately.[21]

In the days after the hijackers' attacks, federal officials were lauded for their efficiency and organization. But during the anthrax crisis, the story was very different. As the *New York Times* put it, "In their initial handling of the anthrax crisis, [federal] government leaders did almost everything wrong." Secretary of Health and Human Services Tommy Thompson, who had little credibility on health matters, was designated the spokesperson on anthrax rather than the director of the CDC or a senior doctor at the National Institutes of Health; and "health and law enforcement authorities made confident statements that later proved false, tried simultaneously to inform and reassure, and limited the flow of information to the public." The *Times* cited one of Thompson's "most egregious lapses": he said that the initial anthrax victim might have contracted the disease by drinking water from a stream in North Carolina.[22] Matters improved when Anthony Fauci, director of the National Institute of Allergy and Infectious Diseases, began taking charge of communicating with the public.

In short, the responses to 9/11 and to the anthrax mailings highlighted some of greatest assets of the public health infrastructure: "9/11 revealed the strengths in individual people" and the much-maligned civil servants who maintain the system, remembers Steven Rubin, deputy director for sexually transmitted diseases, one of the programs of the city's Department of Health directly involved in responding to bioterrorism. He adds, "So many people in this agency responded so quickly and put in so many dedicated hours." The events "revealed the real strengths of the public health infrastructure . . . in that most people came in the next day, the day after, and just showed their commitment to doing the job."[23] But they also illuminated some of the department's most glaring weaknesses and profound needs — to train doctors, nurses, police, and firefighters in bioterrorism emergency response; to expand laboratory capacities sufficiently to handle possible surges in demand; to improve methods of communicating information to emergency personnel; and to maintain the facilities required (including a supply of beds) to cope with a possible emergency.

SCIENTIFIC UNCERTAINTY AND PUBLIC HEALTH COMMUNICATION

Over the weeks and months following the World Trade Center attack, failure to keep New Yorkers informed led to a severe breakdown in public trust, as ambiguous, often contradictory information was communicated and miscommunicated to residents near the WTC site, undocumented workers responsible for cleaning nearby buildings, and parents of children who attended neighborhood elementary, intermediate, and high schools—notably Public School (P.S.) 89, P.S. 150, P.S. 190, P.S. 234, P.S. 875, Intermediate School (I.S.) 289, and the High School for Leadership and Public Service. The case of Stuyvesant High School, one of the elite public schools in the city and indeed the nation, is particularly revealing, as officials and public health experts failed to acknowledge uncertainty and therefore confused the public by sending incoherent messages. Stuyvesant is located five blocks north of the WTC, and most of the students witnessed the planes crashing into the buildings and people jumping and falling from the towers before their collapse.

Stuyvesant High School

David Klasfeld, deputy chancellor for operations at the New York City Board of Education, vividly recalls the confusion and uncertainty that marked the first moments following the attack. He watched the scene from his office at 110 Livingston Street in downtown Brooklyn, and then with Chancellor Harold O. Levy; and the administrators at the Board of Education were unsure of what to do. As they met with the chancellor, they raised questions that had never before been addressed. Should the board send all 1.1 million children home from school? No, because doing so would undoubtedly create mass confusion and panic among hundreds of thousands of parents at work and unable to get to their children, who would therefore be wandering the streets alone. Should it order the schools around the WTC site to evacuate? to send the children in a particular direction? to stay in place?

"I don't believe that we were immediately in contact with [the principals]," Klasfeld says.

The actions of the principals and the teachers in those schools was extraordinary. Remember, this is September 11. . . . It's the third day of school, the fourth day of school. Some of these people are teaching for the first time. It's their third day of work, their fourth day of work. Many of them are young. The board is not one of these places that encourages people to think their own thoughts about what to do. The evacuation plan for those schools south of the World Trade Center was to go north. That was the plan. Instead, they had the sense to go south. North was where danger was.

The board was far away from the scene, leaving the central administration feeling completely helpless, and even at the scene itself principals were at a loss. "You didn't know what to do."[24]

Yet individual principals and teachers took initiative. The High School for Leadership and Public Service, on Trinity Place just below the Twin Towers, moved its children to Battery Park, safe from the falling buildings. "The [most] amazing story to me," declares Klasfeld,

is the woman who is the principal of Leadership, a woman named Ada Rosario Dolch, whose sister died in one of the buildings. She certainly knew that [her sister] was working there. She takes her kids south, puts them on whatever ferry is there — ferry to New Jersey, ferry to Staten Island — gets them off the island. [She] sends teachers with them. There were kids overnight in New Jersey. Cannot get in touch with the chancellor's office, and walks. The only thing on her mind was to tell the chancellor that her kids were OK. She and her secretary and one other walk from Lower Manhattan across the Brooklyn Bridge to 110 Livingston Street, so she can report to the chancellor that she got her kids out.

The staffs of the city's schools were on their own, and in the weeks ahead the board would find that its personnel were in some cases truly heroic. Security personnel, custodians, and other employees played crucial roles in maintaining the schools following their abandonment. Klasfeld points out,

Our custodians, our much-maligned custodians, stayed on the sites of their schools. A number of them, particularly the custodian at Stuyvesant, did a fabulous job. He immediately turned off all of the air systems, so that debris was not sucked into the school at Stuyvesant. . . . One of the issues [that the custodians were concerned about] was nothing that I would ever think about. . . . If it rained, it would be a big problem with the roofs of these buildings. You had all of the ash and stuff. If it rained, then it hardened. So we had our custodians on roofs cleaning off debris, so that that wouldn't happen. So we had our own people at the schools responsible for protecting them.

Immediately after the disaster, and after the children were evacuated, Stuyvesant was taken over by emergency workers and made unavailable for school use. Classes for the students resumed less than a week later at Brooklyn Technical High School in split sessions with shortened class periods. Initially, many parents mobilized to press for an early return to Stuyvesant's very modern and technologically advanced building, arguing that it was important for the children to resume their normal routines. The parents, many of whom were among the city's most sophisticated professionals, including a good number of lawyers and doctors, recognized from the start that health hazards might be present; they hired their own experts to evaluate the safety of the school, which the city planned to reopen on October 9, less than a month after the attack. The city also was intent on returning the students to other schools in the area as quickly as possible.

The city began testing for asbestos, lead, and other toxins and concluded that the air within the building was safe. It hired two eighty-person crews to vacuum air ducts, replace carpets, hose down the ten-story building, and clean all surfaces. In addition, it installed monitoring devices to sample the air quality on a regular basis.[25]

David Klasfeld recalls the heated emotions that engulfed the Board of Education and "wary Stuyvesant parents [who] have enlisted their own experts to determine if the school is safe." Parents began to worry as they heard reports of asbestos-laden dust samples in P.S. 150, a few blocks away; moreover, dust samples taken by the EPA right outside Stuyvesant on September 19 found above-normal levels of asbestos. The city, and particularly Mayor Giuliani, claimed that the tests, with the exception of a few idiosyncratic results, showed that "the air quality [was] safe and acceptable." Parents, however, began to argue that the individual samples were not outliers but reflected a reality obvious to anyone who visited the area and smelled the air: whatever the readings, the smell alone indicated that the air was dangerous for the children.[26]

The students reentered Stuyvesant on Tuesday, October 9, with a mixture of fear and excitement.[27] But students looking out a north window soon noticed huge barges, less than a hundred yards away, carrying debris from the WTC site to the Fresh Kills landfill on Staten Island. Dump trucks carrying WTC debris continuously traveled right past the school, and large plumes of dust covered the bridge that connected Stuyvesant to Chambers Street. As one parent put it, walking to school was like "walking through a construction site." Children likened it to a war zone.[28] At the Stuyvesant High School Parents' Association meeting in November, angry parents were assured by Board of Education officials that all was safe and that virtually all tests for lead and asbestos, the two substances regularly monitored, showed levels well below acceptable standards.

But rumors began circulating among the students themselves that they were all being poisoned, and some began to stay home from class. In the ensuing days and weeks, parents noticed that their children were developing bronchitis, asthma, rashes, coughs, and tremendous anxiety. Children came home with watering eyes and coughs.[29] "I've had bronchitis for the past two weeks. . . . Everyone's coughing," one student observed. Some students wore paper masks to school, and the New York *Daily News* reported that nearly half of the respondents to its informal poll had "some kind of health complaint."[30] While parents and some in the popular press began to conclude that Stuyvesant and the surrounding schools were unsafe, the Board of Education and its experts argued that none of the tests gave any indication of possible danger to the children at Stuyvesant and other local schools. "All the tests showed that the [Stuyvesant] building is safe," commented Jacqueline Moline of Mt. Sinai School of Medicine.[31] The only problem that could be documented was slightly elevated levels of carbon dioxide.[32]

The distance between the parents and the Board of Education kept growing. In large measure the board depended on expert opinion and air monitoring as the basis for declaring Stuyvesant High School safe, while parents relied on their own senses and on those of their children, many of whom were experiencing a variety of symptoms, as they questioned the safety of the environment in and around the school. Throughout the winter and spring, new studies that appeared — far from reassuring parents — served only to fuel the distrust. A CDC study in May 2002 documented that "more than half the employees at Stuyvesant High School suffered respiratory problems after returning to their school on the edge of ground zero in October." Teachers in the school told of their own anxieties, describing what they had "put [their] bodies through." And many complained of depression and high levels of anxiety in addition to physical illness. Twenty-three percent of the staff showed signs of possible post-traumatic stress disorder.[33]

Before the end of 2001, a reshuffling of the parents' association brought in new leaders who more readily accepted the official test results; but other parents formed a new organization, whose members picketed outside the school and called for more and better tests. The board's reassurances were seriously undermined when extremely high readings for asbestos were found in the auditorium, where students, faculty, and parents regularly met.[34] The conflict continued into the next school year, which began twelve months after the attacks.

The struggle over Stuyvesant came to symbolize a larger battle over who should have the authority to judge the long-term health impact of the 9/11 attacks. A variety of pressures from the city, state, and federal bureaucracy to return Lower Manhattan to something approaching a normal state collided with the public's continuing sense of anxiety as well as individuals' everyday perceptions of the local environment. David Klasfeld recalls the implicit and explicit pressure that came from numerous sources, but most directly from the mayor's office: "There was enormous effort on behalf of the mayor, the governor, the president, to return to normalcy as quickly as possible, so that it was moved from 14th Street to Canal Street, the parts of the city that were open, and then Canal Street, further down. Again, schools, as part of the infrastructure of the city, are important and seen as an important component of normalcy. So there was this push to sort of reopen those schools that we could, as soon as we could."

Expert opinion in this case served neither to resolve the scientific issues nor to allay the fears of those who worked, lived, or went to school in the area. In fact, one victim of the struggle between the Board of Education and the parents was the authority of science itself. In the months after the initial school crisis, a much broader debate about environmental health and the dangers posed by contaminants arose, and it fundamentally challenged how danger and risk were understood. After the catastrophe at ground zero, officials from the EPA and other agencies immediately sought to reassure populations who lived, worked, and went to school in the area that the environment, particularly the air, was safe. Depending largely on tools, instruments, and ideas developed to assess dangers to workers in industrial environments — the nation's factories, mines, and mills — experts and officials took air samples, gauged the size of asbestos particles, and measured the amount of lead, then compared the results to the known threshold limits.

But statements that values were below the acceptable thresholds did little to silence the growing complaints of those whose children came home from school with coughs, watering eyes, and burning lungs, and their protests ultimately forced the officials and scientists to reevaluate their tools, instruments, and assumptions about the applicability of their science to this completely new and unexpected experience. Barbara Aaron, director of many 9/11 projects at the Department of Epidemiology at Columbia University's Mailman School of Public Health, notes the profound rift that led many to distrust official pronouncements and even government itself. Indeed, she calls the actions of the city "a terrible political mistake and betrayal." She continues, "Even if you think of it in the most clinical terms, it was such a mistake. Probably morally, it's terrible to pretend to know what you don't know, and say things are OK when they're not. To send children back to school in a toxic environment. But I think that politically, how dumb do you think [people] are? I don't believe that there were terrible poisons everywhere. But I do believe that crushed gypsum and concrete and dust in the air made people really, really sick and contaminated their lungs. . . . The fact that it wasn't acknowledged was really terrible."[35]

The Neighborhood around the WTC

In the aftermath of 9/11, the workers cleaning up the site as well as residents and merchants in the neighborhood around the WTC were potentially exposed to a wide range of dangers. For the Department of Health and specifically for Kelly McKinney in Regulatory and Environmental Health Services, the immediate concerns centered on the possibility that the attack might have released radioactive materials (from the airplanes and the buildings) into the air. The department sent "two of our inspectors down there with radiation-detection equipment so that they could see whether there had been a release of radiation" from the planes, from dentists' and doctors' offices in the area, and particularly from X-ray machines.

For weeks after the attack, McKinney's unit focused on providing proper respiratory equipment for the workers involved in rescue and recovery efforts at the site, though the data he was accumulating indicated that the workforce was in greater danger from accidents and injuries on the job than from the air. Even so, McKinney recalls, "We wanted them to be in respirators, and we pushed for respirators. . . . We knew there was a lot of stuff in the air. I would never say that the air quality was good down there, because it wasn't." But the science led him to believe that it presented no immediate danger. "We had [a] big problem. Because the data looked good, we wanted to communicate the risks but we didn't really want to communicate the data per se, because the data was so good a lot of savvy workers would say, 'Look, if the data is that good, why do I have to wear a respirator?'" The policy seemed incoherent. On the one hand, the department thought it prudent for workers to use respirators; on the other hand, the substances being tested for did not exceed accepted safety levels. (Over the next year, it became clear that even if toxins were not present at dangerous levels, other substances in the air posed serious health risks to workers at the Trade Center site.)

For about two months following the attacks, environmental and health officials in the New York City Department of Health and at the federal EPA and Occupational Safety and Health Administration (OSHA) insisted that "there were no indications of serious long-term health risks" to residents of downtown Manhattan.[36] The city's Department of Health stated that "the general public's risk for any short or long term adverse health [effects is] extremely low," and EPA Administrator Christine Todd Whitman declared, "There's no need for the general public to be concerned."[37] Both agencies had developed what they presented as "an intricate network of tests, standards, and procedures that they said were intended to ensure the safety of those working at the site as well as those living and working in Lower Manhattan."[38] According to the *New York Times,* Jessica Leighton, assistant commissioner for environmental risk assessment in New York's Department of Health, noted that "while tests had recorded occasional spikes in the levels of various contaminants, including asbestos, at some locations at or near the site, long-term health risks are associated with consistent exposure over a 30-year period."[39] But such reassurances were often unpersuasive, even to the professionals in nearby city offices.

In fact, the story was much more complex. Confusion about the meaning of scientific data was compounded by "complete bureaucratic bungling," in the words of U.S. Representative Jerrold Nadler, whose district encompasses the World Trade Center. Nadler speaks emotionally about what he calls the "illegal actions" of the EPA in refusing to implement the National Contingency Plan (NCP) of the Comprehensive Environmental Response, Compensation and Liability Act. The Superfund Act, as it is more commonly known, would have put the EPA in charge of indoor as well as outdoor cleanup. Nadler argues that the release of chemicals "should have triggered the NCP, which should have given the EPA immense powers. The EPA can enter any premise with no warning in order to inspect and decontaminate." Instead, the EPA (and the State Department of Environmental Protection) referred to the New York City Department of Health those residents who asked whether it was appropriate to move back into their apartments and how to clean them. The Department of Health, in turn, foisted responsibility for the decision to move back onto apartment dwellers themselves. Further, according to Nadler, the department suggested that residents clean their homes with "a damp cloth," advice Nadler condemned as "reckless and illegal."[40]

In late October and early November, as residents began to return to their homes to inspect damage, and as the schools reopened and Wall Street businesses and the New York Stock Exchange sought to return to normal, public perceptions began to seriously conflict with official pronouncements. On October 26, 2001, Juan Gonzalez of the *Daily News* published the first in a series of articles that challenged the claims being made by city, state, and federal officials and disseminated by the *New York Times*. In an article titled "A Toxic Nightmare at Disaster Site," Gonzalez drew on EPA documents to charge that "dioxins, PCBs, benzene, lead, and chromium are among the toxic substances detected in the air and soil around the WTC site by Environmental Protection Agency equipment — sometimes at levels far exceeding federal standards." Well into October, benzene levels were between sixteen and fifty-eight times higher than OSHA's permissible limit.[41] Local political representatives, including Representative Nadler and New York City Council Member Kathryn Freed, started to give voice to local residents' concerns and held hearings about the environmental impact of 9/11. At issue was the growing distance between the scientific measurements that had become the bedrock for official pronouncements of safety and New Yorkers' personal experience with the coughs, colds, and smells that accompanied the cleanup. One community board member put it bluntly: "Just because [the measurement of a given contaminant] doesn't reach a certain level is really irrelevant when people are sick."[42]

By November, residents' private doubts were emerging as very public issues. New York City Council Member Stanley Michels, chair of the council's Committee on Environmental Protection, held a hearing that "raised more questions than it answered." Sounding a theme that would become pervasive in subsequent months, he said that "the various tests and standards . . . may be fine for things that have happened in the past, but we don't know if it applies here because the situation is so unique." He recognized the need to keep residents and workers from panicking, yet he qualified his statements by arguing that such reassurances could be given only "if the confidence is due. But the jury's still out on that."[43]

In late November, the *Daily News* reported that according to EPA officials and "public health experts," "government agencies monitoring the air quality near Ground Zero had lost much of their credibility with the public." Their "argument that the air is safe is not registering with the public — particularly those who have felt irritation from smoke and dust near Ground Zero." George Thurston, an environmental scientist from New York University's School of Medicine, worried that reliance on the measurements was undermining the credibility of the science itself, while

Philip Landrigan of the Mt. Sinai School of Medicine was concerned about misuse of the data he and others were collecting: "Risk communication is more than spin. If you think it's spin, then you've lost the battle already." Increasingly, the scientific community tried to introduce subtle distinctions that were lacking in declarations from the political establishment. Thus Thurston summarized the scientific evidence: "I think it is premature to tell people it is safe, but we can tell people we don't see a danger." Madelyn Wills, chair of Community Board 1, drew the opposite conclusion: "The air may not be toxic, but the air is not safe. There is a distinction here," she argued, because, for example, residents of Lower Manhattan were experiencing marked increases in rates of asthma.[44]

Government officials had initially concentrated on the lack of danger from exposure at ground zero, but their argument shifted in November and December as they began to distinguish between the short-term and long-term health effects of breathing the air and absorbing toxins. Though the immediate effects of exposure were obvious — increased congestion, tearing eyes, and headaches — they were, officials insisted, also temporary, and the long-term impact was negligible. Only those with existing respiratory problems or asthma need worry about any serious damage to their health, if the contact was brief.[45] The scientific community was doing what it could to document the possible dangers long recognized by environmental and occupational physicians, and, by and large, its findings were at worst troubling and at best mildly reassuring. But since only a few air samples showed elevated levels of known toxins such as asbestos and lead, many public officials pronounced the environment around the WTC site acceptable.

The Need for New Methods of Evaluating Environmental Hazards

Some scientists began to suggest that a new framework was needed to understand the health effects of this disaster. First, Stephen Levin, medical director of the Mt. Sinai–Irving J. Selikoff Center for Occupational and Environmental Medicine, claimed that the older techniques for evaluating danger might not suffice for this new situation. Second, he argued that the residents' complaints could not be easily dismissed, regardless of the tests' results. Coughs, nosebleeds, and respiratory ailments were being triggered by the dust and debris in the air. He declared, "This wasn't about breathing dust" — that is, tiny particles. "It was breathing chunks of material." Standards had been developed for specific chemicals but few if any existed for measuring the impact of the variety and inter-actions of chemical materials released in the burning and collapse of a hundred-story building. One industrial hygienist complained that scientists were "not looking at the incredible number of plasticizers, fire retardants, fillers. You have 210 floors of carpets, wallboard, furniture and computers burning. We have no idea what this will do."[46]

Thirty thousand gallons of transformer fluids containing PCBs, 180,000 gallons of fuel, hundreds of thousands of fluorescent bulbs each containing small amounts of mercury, and millions of pounds of other toxins introduced a level of uncertainty that the scientific apparatus for measuring lead and asbestos could not even begin to evaluate.[47] One reporter for the London *Guardian* likened the effect to that of "a major explosion in a giant chemical works," with "thousands of tons of pulverized asbestos and heavy metals . . . leaving an estimated 2m[illion] cubic meters of dust covering [16 acres]."[48] A major problem was the inadequacy of the scientific tools traditionally used to gauge danger. Threshold limits for dangerous substances were established for industrial workers, assumed to be exposed for eight hours a day. "The permissible levels for asbestos, for example," says Ekaterina Malievskaia of Queens College's Center for the Biology of Natural Systems, "are based on linear extrapolation from effects resulting from heavy occupational exposure in the past. These risk estimates are highly uncertain." And even those estimates were generally understood to be guidelines rather than hard-and-fast standards. "There are essentially no conclusive prospective human studies on the safe levels of [environmental] exposure," she continues.[49]

Unions, tenant groups, contractors, and New York political leaders hired independent scientists and physicians — many of whom had served in the past as consultants to the EPA — whose tests revealed much higher levels of toxins than the official results. One newspaper described their approach: "Taking hundreds of samples, many inside apartments, offices, and condos, these experts used the newest electron microscope technology and fiber-counting protocols" and found levels of asbestos comparable to those at the Superfund site of Libby, Montana. One EPA scientist said, "It is unfathomable to believe that EPA can stand behind antiquated science when the report on Libby, issued by the same agency, irrefutably documents the validity of the new methods." While the Department of Health told residents that "asbestos-related lung disease results only from intense asbestos exposure experienced over a period of many years, primarily as a consequence of occupational exposures," EPA and CDC experts acknowledged a different reality. Their research had shown that "a 'single burst, heavy dose' of asbestos could be enough to cause lethal disease."[50]

Steven Markowitz of Queens College's Center for the Biology of Natural Systems lamented, "What's most striking to me [is] that I can't begin to answer [basic] questions. . . . For all the thousands of air quality samples, here we are eight months out and there's such limited health data." The problem arose in large part, as the *New York Times* reported, because many substances created in the WTC disaster "had never been seen in nature or in the laboratory. Metals and glass from windows and computers and girders were turned into mist by the intense heat and pressure of the collapse, and those mist particles then bonded with larger pieces of concrete, creating billions of tiny hybrid fragments, each coated with a sheath created from the elements of destruction. Asbestos was pulverized into pieces so tiny that ordinary tests devised to track the fibers missed them."[51]

By early February 2002, according to the *Times*, about three-quarters of the 20,000-odd people who lived within half a mile of the site had returned to their homes.[52] Yet local and federal agencies had done little testing of the air quality within the apartments, and even those tests had not been made available to the residents or the public.[53] At congressional hearings held by Jerrold Nadler in February, the agencies found themselves under intense pressure and scrutiny as their assurances of safety and efficiency were rejected. The day following the hearings, the State Department of Environmental Protection (DEP) sent out notices to landlords to "clean up the public areas of their buildings." But they did not require landlords to clean up apartments or ventilation systems. Also, the state allowed landlords to "self-certify" their own work.[54] At a subsequent hearing, Nadler reports, the DEP head argued that "the insides of the buildings had been cleaned" and, according to Nadler, "the entire room, four hundred people, erupted in laughter."

"There was no government database, no handy list of indoor air monitors to pull down from a website" that would tell returning residents whether or not their apartments were safe. The Natural Resources Defense Council reported that "because no one government agency was in charge of the overall environmental impact . . . issues of residential indoor air quality fell between the cracks, and because of the emphasis on long-term risks, the impact on susceptible populations was not emphasized enough." The cleanup inside the buildings was left "to building owners and managers — some of whom might have had an interest in minimizing the risk, or have limited resources to clean what they found."[55] Largely neglected in the months following the event was the inspection and decontamination of office buildings and apartments in the area. Finally, in May 2002, the EPA accepted responsibility for inspecting homes below Canal Street;[56] but by then this response was deemed inadequate by Nadler's office and residents in the area, as well as others outside it. Trust had dissolved, as Nadler explains, and suspicions about the limited scope of the EPA's efforts abounded. Nadler himself attacked the EPA for ignoring residents above Canal Street and for focusing only on asbestos, not other materials, in its testing and remediation. "The agencies have [sought to leave] the impression in the public's mind that it's safer than it really is," claimed Joel Kupferman, director of the New York Environmental Law and Justice Project. "This whole thing about returning to normalcy has gone too far."[57]

Protecting Undocumented Workers

Great care was taken to protect as fully as possible the workers clearing ground zero, but those hired to clean up private residences and other office buildings in the area were given less consideration. Right after September 11, there was a determined effort to reopen the Stock Exchange as part of the broader policy to return Lower Manhattan to "normal" and to stabilize the city's and the nation's financial sector — an agenda that often came into conflict with health issues. Ekaterina Malievskaia, a physician who worked with the Latin American Workers' Project at the scene in the months following the attack, recalls the drive to "open up Wall Street," noting that "one of the [cleaning companies] told me that in the beginning . . . they employed up to 1,800 day laborers for cleaning purposes. It's just one corporation. And there were about thirty major cleaning companies involved in efforts to clean up [the buildings] around ground zero." She describes how the companies recruited their workforce: "They got all these illegal immigrants on every corner [of the city] and they threw them into the buildings and gave them rags and sometimes paper masks and that's it. They cleaned for twelve, fourteen hours a day without any protection, without knowing what they were exposed to. And Wall Street got opened on time. So it worked out in a sense."[58]

Not only were the workers hired and thrust into dangerous jobs indiscriminately, but companies actually went out of their way to deny workers adequate protection. Malievskaia relates that some of the workers had earlier received licenses to remove asbestos, since for undocumented laborers this is one of the few avenues to relatively high-paying jobs. Asbestos removal, she explains, "is a dirty job that Americans don't want to do, and [trade schools] don't ask whether you're legal or illegal." When these trained workers, who had their own respirators, were cleaning buildings near ground zero, "they were asked not to wear these respirators by the employers so they wouldn't scare the rest of their co-workers off." Those who sought to use their own respirators "were not given filters. And if they had a couple of filters [of their own] and kept on reusing them, it [made] things even worse," because the used filters would become a repository for dangerous materials that the worker ultimately breathed in.

By December 2001, the danger to the day laborers hired by private companies to clean apartments and offices was becoming a public issue. The New York Committee for Occupational Safety and Health joined with the Latin American Workers' Project and the Center for the Biology of Natural Systems at Queens College to identify and evaluate the health effects of the cleanup effort on the hundreds of nonunion and largely undocumented workers hired to clean buildings. The groups approached the New York Community Trust and the September 11th Fund for money to undertake the study. "It was an incredible turnaround . . . about three weeks" between submission and funding for such a screening project. Initially, according to Malievskaia, the methods of identifying World Trade Center cleanup workers were informal and often haphazard. "In the beginning [the workers] heard the announcement on the radio. But what got the program going was the word of mouth. They told their neighbors, workers. It's the nature of their job that they shape up on the corners, and while they're standing in line waiting for jobs they have nothing to talk about other than just describe the program . . . and it was, you know, a great demand." They had originally hoped to "serve 150 to 200 people," she recalls, but they ended up seeing more than 400 workers.[59]

The workers had been put in an insupportable position. As Steven Markowitz, the head of the project, put it, they "were looking down on ground zero, seeing people wearing respirators, and they're working indoors in a confined space, and they don't have them."[60] By May, the Queens College Center had uncovered nearly universal respiratory and systemic health problems; symptoms included difficulty in breathing, nasal congestion, coughs, headaches, difficulty in sleeping, and numbness.[61] A year later, as noted above, the EPA agreed to take over responsibility for cleaning apartments and other buildings in the area. Even today, arguments about the possible health effects suffered by workers, students, and local residents exposed to various contaminants from the WTC site continue.

In rushing to normalcy, the government had not waited to gather evidence before reassuring citizens that ground zero and the community around it were safe. Hence, schoolchildren, residents, and workers were put at risk. In August 2003, the EPA Office of Inspector General issued an "evaluation report" that concluded that at the time when the EPA had announced — a week after the attack — "that the air was 'safe' to breathe, it did not have sufficient data and analyses to make such a blanket statement. At that time, air monitoring data was lacking for several pollutants of concern, including particulate matter and polychlorinated biphenyls (PCBs)." Moreover, the report criticized the White House Council on Environmental Quality for shaping the agency's recommendations, influencing "the information that EPA communicated to the public through its early press releases when it convinced EPA to add reassuring statements and delete cautionary ones." Thus, only years later did the EPA admit what critics had insisted at the time: "A definitive answer to whether the air was safe to breathe may not be settled for years to come." Rather than give in to those with whom it collaborates, the "EPA needs to be prepared to assert its opinion and judgment on matters that impact human health and the environment." Although the report determined that the EPA had not violated any regulations in ceding authority to local authorities, it suggested that the "EPA could have taken a more proactive approach regarding indoor air clean-up." Despite the repeated demands of local community groups, better and more accurate information was late in coming.[62]

This acknowledgment of the EPA's shortcomings stimulated further discussion of the federal government's actions in the weeks and months following the attack. In August 2004, the Sierra Club issued a comprehensive report — titled "Air Pollution (and Deception) at Ground Zero" — that details how the EPA and other federal agencies "failed to take important actions after the attack to prevent more exposures to contaminants. . . . Independent researchers found a group of toxic pollutants that cause cancer and other genetic effects, while EPA wrongly claimed that it did not detect the presence of these pollutants at all. . . . The federal administration's reckless disregard for the toxic hazards generated by the attack had disastrous consequences for many people who served on the front line of terror response in Lower Manhattan's recovery."[63]

SOCIAL SERVICES

The Immediate Relief Effort

Much as the experience of 9/11 challenged assumptions about risk and how to measure it, its aftermath presented a tremendous test for the voluntary social service agencies that traditionally have had the responsibility of caring and providing for the city's dependent and poor. Thousands of large and small agencies, churches, community groups, foundations, and individuals poured time and money into the relief and recovery effort. This vast charitable enterprise, which won wide praise for its inclusiveness and the breadth of services provided, was also notable because it implicitly challenged the existing social service model, which required that strict criteria be established to determine who should receive benefits.

Our analysis of social services is divided into two broad categories: the short-term responses to the crisis and the longer-term impact of 9/11 on how services are organized. In the short term, 9/11 highlighted the sector's extraordinary ability to mobilize and distribute resources to the immediate victims of the attack and to populations throughout the city whose lives were grievously altered or disrupted. In the long term, certain assumptions that have traditionally dominated the delivery of social and mental health services were seriously challenged.

One major weakness was revealed in the wake of September 11 when the thousands of frail and disabled people who lived below Canal Street and even in the rest of Manhattan found themselves without assistance. In the immediate aftermath of the tragedy, many workers who provided services to the homebound in the downtown area could not get to their clients. "A lot of the home care workers who go into people's homes don't live in the ground zero area," points out Igal Jellinek, executive director of the Council of Senior Centers and Services of New York City. "So there was a blockade, you couldn't get through. There was no system of photo identification, of how to get in and out."[64] Representative Jerrold Nadler recalls that "there were seven hundred senior citizens trapped in Southbridge Houses, just below the Brooklyn Bridge. They couldn't get food in or their prescriptions in. . . . In fact, all the pharmacies were closed, so they had to arrange for a runner and get one of the pharmacies open. Then they had to get the governor to waive the public health provision that says the pharmacy can't fill a prescription" without verbal or written instructions from a physician. Patients themselves were the authority when coming to the pharmacy. Nadler helped set up the Ground Zero Elected Officials Task Force, which assisted in fulfilling these needs for local residents and thereby helped relieve the already overburdened communication system.

Elsewhere in Manhattan, the Meals on Wheels program was crippled because, as Jellinek noted, "the trucks that brought in the food were stuck out in Queens, with the bridges and tunnels shut down."[65] The social service agencies had to scramble to find alternatives. For example, food for the Stanley Isaacs Senior Center on the Upper East Side was normally brought in from Queens, but the normal procedure was now impossible. In that case, says Jellinek, "What they did is they went to some of the fanciest restaurants on the East Side, who really came through for them and prepared the meals and helped them deliver" the food to the elderly residents.

As Jellinek explained to a special committee of the U.S. Senate, being cut off from the usual deliveries was not just a nutritional issue but quickly became "an emotional one as well, as isolation, fear, and panic set in, all with terrible consequences for the homebound person." Thus, while closing down the bridges and tunnels may have been important for safety reasons, "it sent senior services providers without local emergency backup scrambling to cover the necessities that we took for granted before the attack of 9/11." As a result of that scrambling, the elderly clients had to come to senior centers and other "congregate facilities" because of their need "to be in touch with someone — anyone — to stave off the terror of isolation amid a disaster of such earthshaking proportion." In the experience of 9/11, Jellinek found five lessons for the social service community, which needed to get "services to the homebound and the disabled"; to ensure that "seniors have adequate food, water, and shelter"; to ensure "adequate transportation" of people, services, medications, and food; to guarantee "360-degree communications with staff, seniors, their families, and emergency organizations"; and to take care to address "the mental health issues that arise for everyone."[66]

Interestingly, at times the roles of clients and staff were reversed, as some of the seniors had lived through disasters and wars and were able to put the events of September 11 into a larger perspective. Jellinek remembers that "some of the seniors were coping very well" with the emotional anguish that affected most New Yorkers. When he called one center in Jamaica, Queens, he found that "the seniors were comforting the staff."

Private Aid and Public Needs

Because 9/11 occasioned such an immense relief effort, it highlighted major problems in how to handle the outpouring of giving that ensued. The instant response to September 11 was a flood of assistance by individual agencies that provided money, shelter, food, and social services to the families immediately affected by the disaster.[67] Most of that money went to the American Red Cross, but it also was directed to the Twin Towers Fund (for families of rescuers who died), the Uniformed Firefighters Association's Widows and Children's Fund, the New York Times 9/11 Neediest Fund, and dozens of smaller social service agencies. The effort on behalf of the smaller agencies was soon coordinated by the September 11th Fund, an organization started by the New York Community Trust and United Way of New York City. As of March 1, 2002, the fund had made 181 grants totaling $205 million to dozens of social service agencies.[68]

Because so many organizations were collecting huge sums of money, politicians and the media were concerned that all the funds might not be used to directly aid the victims of September 11. The largest relief organization, the American Red Cross, came in for harsh criticism when it announced, and later retracted, a policy "not to immediately distribute all of the hundreds of millions of dollars it raised as part of its Sept. 11 response."[69] After accumulating $543 million, the Red Cross had set aside $264 million for its reserves. Further, it had decided to provide only $154 million as direct assistance and put $150 million toward other programs, such as improvements in its system of supplying blood. Its admission that moneys were being socked away for future use came at a time when smaller agencies throughout the city were beginning to complain that their fund-raising was drying up because all the charitable giving was going to September 11 relief, and these actions of the Red Cross were perceived as a gross injustice. New York State Attorney General Eliot Spitzer called the Red Cross's decision to put aside more than half of the moneys gathered for support of programs not directly linked to September 11 "totally unacceptable," adding that it "breaks one's heart to know the funds are there but yet they are not traveling."[70] A week after Spitzer's attack, the Red Cross reversed course, announcing it would spend the entire $543 million fund on the victims themselves as it "apologized to the public for its earlier decision to reserve some of the money for other uses."[71]

Yet the Red Cross had acted in response to what the broader social service community saw as the necessity to plan for the long term as well as to respond to immediate crises. This was a perception that personnel had taken away from the experience of Oklahoma City, where domestic terrorism had destroyed the Alfred P. Murrah Federal Building a few years before. Igal Jellinek describes one discussion at a board meeting of the National Association of Nutrition and Aging Services Programs that took place a few weeks after that attack, during which one member from Oklahoma "kept telling us, 'Don't spend all your money up front,' because there's long-range ramifications and there's all sorts of issues that are going to come up. In Oklahoma a lot of money was spent early and therefore there wasn't the money" later to address the long-term mental health and social service needs that began to emerge.

The outpouring of money and effort, haphazard as it might have been, was effective in addressing the immediate needs of most families of those killed at the World Trade Center. But as the Red Cross imbroglio soon made clear, there were different definitions of what constituted "assistance." Some saw it as the provision of cash and cash substitutes to the families of victims for rent, food, clothing, and other necessities. Others took a much broader view, arguing that a portion of the money should be set aside to support long-term mental health services and to develop the public health infrastructure.

By December 2001, it was becoming apparent that the various agencies' lack of coherent aims and their inability to set joint priorities were hurting the long-term relief effort. Although the city's various charities and social service agencies are coordinated at least nominally through the efforts of Jewish, Protestant, and Catholic umbrella organizations as well as the United Way, a new organization was formed — the 9/11 United Services Group (USG), with Robert J. Hurst of Goldman Sachs as its CEO — with the sole purpose of planning and coordinating future activities. Its chief program officer, Jack Krauskopf, notes that it was intended to oversee "the social service agencies that [were] assisting people affected by September 11." In addition to the Salvation Army and American Red Cross, other organizations forming the backbone of the USG included the Asian American Federation, the Hispanic Federation, Black Agency Executives, United Neighborhood Houses, Safe Horizon, the Mental Health Association, and the Human Services Council. Initially started with a seed grant from the September 11th Fund, the new organization, according to Krauskopf, had a mission of working with "social service agencies [to help] them to be more effective in serving people [and] to cooperate better than they otherwise might have."[72]

Attempts to Coordinate Services

Eliot Spitzer brought together a number of the major charities and asked them to establish a database to track the moneys that were coming in and going out. Two and a half weeks after the attacks, Spitzer criticized Bernadine Healy, president of the American Red Cross, for statements that her agency "would not share information with other agencies on people it had helped, out of concern for their privacy," and he sought the Red Cross's "help with [the] proposed database."[73] The lack of coordination among the agencies and the growing suspicion that supposed privacy concerns veiled resistance to oversight increased pressure on the organization until, at the end of October, the Red Cross reversed its policy and opened up its records to the attorney general. The *New York Times* applauded the efforts to "create a database of charitable organizations as well as a companion database of victims."[74]

On December 15 Spitzer joined others in announcing that with the aid of IBM and other large New York firms, a shared database would be created; the 9/11 USG would run it and coordinate services to victims.[75] The USG established a service coordinator network and worked on ways to share information and integrate training for new staff and to improve technology. In particular, it sought to centralize the process of applying for aid to ease the burden on clients who previously were forced to travel from agency to agency to match their needs with a specific agency's goals. Immediately after 9/11, Krauskopf explains, "each agency operated fairly independently, and while it was great that a lot of services and assistance was given, it wasn't given as efficiently or certainly as would be ideal for the kinds of clients and the stress that the people were under in those days."

Private Philanthropy and Long-Term Assistance

The crisis highlighted not only the lack of coordination among the various agencies but also the inadequacy of private philanthropy to cope with the long-term effects of such a massive disaster. According to Jack Krauskopf, the 9/11 USG found "that both the impressive short-term efforts that the agencies had and were making to assist people and the need to respond to longer-term needs for employment assistance, mental health, and other problems were essential."[76] As a 2002 study noted, the agencies recognized that "even the generous $1.5 billion plus in charitable contributions made in response to September 11 represents only a small fraction of the federal government's pledge of tens of billions of dollars in disaster relief. Moreover, the government earmarked hundreds of billions of additional dollars for defense expenditures, internal security measures, and potential economic stimulus provisions to help individuals directly and indirectly affected by the terrorist attacks."[77]

Yet government money could not make up for the vast economic losses. Krauskopf recognized that there were "a lot of needs that aren't being met . . . particularly the economic needs. . . . The number of people that are unemployed or underemployed is well beyond the resources to serve them. And part of that is because there hasn't been as much of a government response to economic needs as there should be." The voluntary agencies provided cash assistance and direct services right after September 11. But "that had to come to an end at some point . . . and the gap has not been picked up by unemployment insurance and FEMA assistance and some of the other forms of government aid that should be there."

The huge amounts of moneys that were pouring in and the nature of the 9/11 tragedy forced a public discussion about who should receive the cash and services that were being provided, the families of victims alone or the broader community of New Yorkers, rich and poor alike, who had been traumatized by the attack — workers at the scene, members of the hastily gathered cleanup crews, children in the schools closest to the WTC, appalled witnesses to the explosions, communities in which the victims lived, communities directly and indirectly affected by the economic impact of the closing of small businesses and services, and undocumented workers whose family members sought aid.[78] A Cleveland newspaper noted the far-reaching issues facing the organizations: "Should charities focus primarily on helping direct victims of the attack even if some are wealthy already and likely to get large payments later from government and private sources? Or should they focus on the neediest people, even if they weren't affected directly by the attacks? Should charities set aside some of the money for future attacks, or should they just assume that Americans will respond as generously if terrorists strike again?"[79]

Even the seemingly obvious method of defining immediate victims by geography was challenged. By June 2002, it became clear that the needs of Manhattan's Chinese community, just a few blocks to the north and east of the WTC site, were being neglected. As the New York Times observed, "Families who live in Battery Park City, where the median household income is $125,000, are eligible for grants of $14,500." But "in Chinatown, where streets were also blocked and garment factories shut after Sept. 11, household income is only a third of that in Tribeca. Yet families there are eligible for grants that reach a maximum of $7,750. The many Chinese families and others in a smaller zone north of Canal Street are eligible for a maximum grant of $1,750."[80]

The attempt to provide relief and support was complicated by the attacks' devastating impact on the economy of Lower Manhattan, and indeed all of New York City. In early 2002 the new mayor, Michael Bloomberg, announced that his proposed budget for the fiscal year 2003 had to address a potential $4 to $5 billion deficit. But as Bloomberg pointed out, the economy had been weakening before 9/11, and the destruction in Lower Manhattan only added to what was already a grim fiscal outlook. From October to December 2001, unemployment in New York City rose by 2.3 percent, almost three times the national increase of 0.8 percent. The WTC disaster was projected to cost the city about $21 billion through June 30, 2002, a figure that did not include the loss of about 115,000 jobs.[81] According to the *New York Times,* the city lost "nearly 80,000 mainly low-income jobs in the month of October alone."[82] Of the 35,500 workers in the twenty-five hardest-hit occupations, 18,000 were in jobs that paid less than $10 an hour; another 10,000 people earned less than $15 an hour, including restaurant workers, janitors and cleaners, maids and housekeepers, sewing machine operators, salesclerks, counter attendants and bartenders, cashiers, and other service workers.[83] Ironically, the loss of jobs and income was felt most severely in Brooklyn, Queens, and the Bronx, not in the neighborhoods closest to the disaster site itself.

Long-Term Problems Exacerbated by 9/11

The effects of 9/11 were made even more severe by the welfare reforms of the 1990s. The Personal Responsibility and Work Opportunity Reconciliation Act (or Welfare Reform Act of 1996) fundamentally changed a sixty-year-old program by effectively limiting the time that families with dependent children could remain on welfare rolls. Welfare eligibility was generally capped at five years over a recipient's lifetime (making October 2001 the termination date for many), and the application process became more onerous for thousands of city residents. By the year 2000, the city's welfare rolls had been reduced by 50 percent, a reduction that saved the state $1.5 billion.

Mimi Abramovitz, professor of social work and social welfare policy at Hunter College School of Social Work, sees this welfare "reform" as an abdication of responsibility by the state and city that forced the city's nonprofit agencies to shift much of "their time and resources away from social services." She concludes, "As New York City's Human Resources Administration has reduced the amount and quality of information and guidance provided to welfare recipients, nonprofit agency staff have had to put aside core service responsibilities in order to help clients understand the new entitlements process." Workers at more than three-quarters of the agencies reported that advocating for their clients was requiring them to devote substantial amounts of their time to talking with public agency representatives by telephone and in person. Workers at food pantries and homeless shelters throughout the city found that their resources were stretched to the limit. Abramovitz notes, "Emergency food providers alone turned away more than 48,000 during 2000. Meanwhile, workers at other agencies are engaged in a continual and often discouraging search for new resources to help an expanding cohort of clients deal with hunger, illness, and homelessness."[84]

Even before September 11, agencies complained that their "workers are running uphill trying to fix the problems created by welfare reform."[85] Welfare experts anticipated that large numbers of clients would be pushed off public assistance, and that some inevitably would find their way to the voluntary services provided by various agencies associated with the United Way, United Jewish Appeal, Federation of Protestant Welfare Agencies, and Catholic Social Services. At the same time, according to a 2001 report, a number of philanthropies were already concerned about their ability to soften the economic downturn's impact, because "the value of their assets had dropped significantly" as the stock market fell. Further, as the recession ate into corporate profits, many companies were "reducing the dollars they could devote to supporting charitable nonprofits" and thereby cutting a major source of support.[86] Because the October deadline coincided with the national recession and the more severe local downturn, local charities expected their caseloads to increase dramatically — particularly since the low-level service jobs that the Welfare Reform Act anticipated would be available to ex-welfare clients were the very jobs most affected by the attack on the World Trade Center.[87]

Igal Jellinek of the Council of Senior Centers and Services notes the complex forces that were unsettling his clients both before and after 9/11. The problems within the city's Department for the Aging (DFTA) were long-standing. In 1980, 77 percent of its budget was provided by the federal government. In 2003, Washington provided 17 percent of that department's budget, now much larger, and New York State provided 6 percent. "The rest is kicked in by the city, and if the city doesn't have money, this is a system that is at risk." Adding to the risk was inconsistent support, both financial and administrative, for social service agencies from the city's DFTA itself. During the Giuliani administration, those in the social service world recognized that the mayor himself appeared to support services for seniors, but that was not enough. As Jellinek puts it, "While the mayor was very supportive of seniors, this support lost some momentum as it worked its way down through the ranks. In other words, money was available, but the voices of seniors and those working with them were not always heard. Today, with the downturn of the economy, budget cuts mean that tough decisions have to be made, and the elderly are not always seen as a priority."[88]

The social welfare community was in crisis not simply because clients lacked income but because they needed housing, food, and health services as well. Most low-income workers had no savings, and those who lost their jobs soon found themselves unable to pay their rent. As the city as a whole had gentrified in the 1990s, the stock of affordable housing available in the outer boroughs, where many of these workers lived, had dropped sharply. The welfare community had to prepare to offer eviction prevention services, financial planning assistance, community mental health services, and support for the thousands of documented and undocumented immigrants not eligible for city aid. The importance of the last is clear when we consider New York's demographics: 40 percent of the population is foreign-born, and this percentage is expected to increase in the coming years. Even before the terrorist attacks, the recession had begun to affect the ability of residents in poor communities to volunteer at local food pantries and shelters. Further, a nonpartisan coalition observed, "food banks have experienced significant drops in corporate food contributions since midsummer [2001], when the first impacts of an economic slowdown were being felt — and at the same time they are experiencing a rapid increase in demand for food supplies."[89]

The impact of the WTC disaster on smaller social service agencies, coming in the midst of a broader crisis caused by the recession and welfare reform, was therefore severe. From soup kitchens to neighborhood clinics, they had few resources and found it difficult to survive, much less expand their services, in the wake of 9/11; larger organizations, in contrast, which had significant cash reserves as well as a broader donor base, often found that their income from various sources remained virtually unaffected but that their priorities had changed. Twenty-five percent of agencies surveyed in one study refocused their efforts on a larger number of outreach programs dedicated to religious tolerance as well as on mental health services and projects addressing the threat of bioterrorism.[90]

The WTC Disaster and the Outer Boroughs

Little of the outpouring of donations for social services and social welfare reached the outer boroughs. At St. Ann's Church in the Mott Haven section of the Bronx, for example, Mother Martha Overall saw her church's food pantry overwhelmed as the numbers of those seeking assistance increased by 30 to 40 percent in October and November 2001. But "outside help was shrinking." She noted that "the charitable donations [following 9/11] went Downtown instead of Uptown."[91] An editorial in the *New York Times* pointed out that "Food for Survival, the city's largest supplier of emergency food, estimated that more than a million New Yorkers were relying on soup kitchens, food pantries, and shelters to avoid going hungry." Although the true extent of dependence on these charity services is difficult to estimate, the New York City Coalition against Hunger also reported a dramatic upsurge in demand.[92]

The city's short-term response to the crisis — providing emergency shelter and support for the families of WTC disaster victims — drew praise as generous and efficient. But one food service provider asked, "Why can't that happen in other times in dealing with poverty?"[93] In October, a business reporter observed the "tremendous concern, verging on panic, among nonprofits not directly related to emergency relief efforts. Most operate with few reserves and uncertain cash-flows. They face an economy that was deteriorating before the attacks and is declining rapidly since; a huge drop in the portfolio values of individuals and foundations, reducing their ability to give; cuts in city and state funding as governments struggle to keep budgets balanced; and the possibility that donors will feel 'tapped out' by giving to disaster relief."[94]

The impact of September 11 on the city's charities has been far-reaching, in ways both concrete and conceptual. The pressures placed on the various agencies led to significant upheavals in the administrative structure of the system as well as a growing theoretical debate about the basis for providing services to individuals and groups. Throughout American history, philanthropies and the government have separated the "worthy" from the "unworthy." Thus, in the Social Security Act of 1935 legislators

distinguished between the elderly, who were in effect automatically enti-
tled to Social Security benefits (Old Age Assistance), and poor single
mothers and their children, who had to prove that they needed and
deserved assistance. These moral distinctions were carried forward into
the Medicare and Medicaid legislation of 1965. But post-9/11, the voluntary sector has begun a vibrant and potentially important discussion of
how one distinguishes between individuals and among groups. In a
thoughtful paper, Eugene Steuerle (writing for the Urban Institute) has
laid out the practical issues that the World Trade Center disaster raised
for large and small voluntary organizations alike. Were benefits to be
given out on the basis of earning potential, or should a principle of hori-
zontal equity be applied? Should resources be given to the most needy or
to all who were affected, irrespective of income? Did charitable agencies
have the right to decide who was most deserving? But hopes that the
response to the immediate crisis would change the basic assumptions
governing who receives care — poor or rich, working or unemployed —
were dashed. As soon as the crisis passed, old distinctions between those
considered worthy and those not resurfaced, once again determining
social policy for the voluntary as well as the public sector.[95]

Mental Health

In the immediate aftermath of the World Trade Center tragedy, the city
responded as generously to mental health as to social needs, providing an
amazing array of services to people without regard for traditional financial or moral criteria. But the experience with mental health highlights
longer-term weaknesses that appear more difficult to overcome than
those in the social service sector, and that may have much more profound
implications for public policy.

Barbara Aaron of Columbia University's Mailman School of Public
Health immediately became involved in attempts to estimate the dimensions of the mental health problems that the city's population would face
in the coming weeks, months, and years. The overwhelming dimensions
of the problems began to emerge as she visited workers at the WTC site.
Several months after the attack she went down into the "pit," now seven
stories below ground. She recalls, "It was a little bit wet in spots but it
was mostly dry . . . and I saw these football-field-size areas, and there
would be a row of men that I realized were firefighters." They were sitting in chairs

sort of slumped, in rows, on either side of this long field, if you will, and a front-haul loader would come and scoop up a big pile of dirt and debris from this huge mountain and would back up between the two rows of men and sift it down, creating an incredible amount of dust in the air. And these guys would sort of heave themselves to their feet, and with rakes and picks and shovels they would just pick through it. And after about ten minutes they would stop and they would sort of slump down in their seats and a bulldozer would come and push it away. And the process would repeat itself endlessly all day.

Aaron describes the physical effects of being in the pit for just a few hours: "My eyes were infected for two weeks after that one day, and I [developed] a really terrible cough. . . . So this [was one of] the cleanest, probably most pristine moments down there, and it was awful. It was loud, it was unpleasant, it smelled bad."

However stressful the physical environment, the emotional strain on the people working in the pit was in some ways worse. Aaron calls it "a grim place, and it was just like the people there were serving some kind of sentence or some kind of penance . . . and this wasn't like a big traumatic moment. But it was very, very grim." When, at a morning meeting at the trailer on-site, she described the services project in which Columbia was engaged, she found that the workers were generally receptive: "They don't say that much, they stare and they nod, and some of them, you know, you see emotion in their faces, and then afterward, they all expressed regret to the guy I was with that they hadn't said more. But they were afraid to say it in front of each other. But people come up and put their arm around you — firefighters come up and say, 'We're OK, but the workers, the workers don't have the support we have. And they do everything we did.' This was a classic response — 'I'm fine, but that guy . . .'"

The Growing Debate about Long-Term Services

Even as a remarkable array of short-term services were being provided by a variety of agencies, institutions, and professional groups, mental health professionals recognized that a substantial proportion of those directly and indirectly affected by the attack would need ongoing and long-term care. In August 2002 the September 11th Fund announced that the provision of mental health services, unlike most social services, would substantively change toward more inclusiveness rather than being primarily needs-based. This shift hints at a series of broader consequences that the response to the crisis may have for health policies at the state and federal levels.

In the days and weeks following September 11 the various health agencies, hospitals, and medical and public health schools established a mental health network to counsel those directly affected. According to a press release from the New York City Department of Mental Health, "Within 24 hours of the World Trade Center collapse, DMH informed the media that its mental health counseling and referral information line — LIFENET — was up and running in English, Spanish, and Asian languages." Staff members were sent to the mayor's Family Assistance Center at Pier 94 and to the morgue.[96]

Throughout the city, different agencies established counseling centers, opening their doors to anyone who came in. Health professionals flooded Lower Manhattan — sometimes to the consternation of officials at ground zero, many of whom told volunteer therapists to go elsewhere. One therapist recalls going to tables set up near the site to organize volunteer professionals; desperately wishing to do something useful, she demanded that she be allowed to "help," even though the people staffing the tables were obviously swamped with offers of aid from scores of other therapists driven by the same impulse.[97] Within two weeks of the event, the New York City DMH had established its own network, offering services at Pier 94, at ground zero, in the Emergency Operations Center at Pier 92, via mental health hotlines, and through 230 community-based mental health agencies throughout the city. The department estimated that it was running 988 programs aimed at providing emergency mental health services for those dealing with "feelings of grief, confusion, and anger" in the weeks after the disaster.[98] The Greater New York Hospital Association's member hospitals, including NYU Downtown Hospital, St. Vincent's, Cabrini, Beth Israel, Mt. Sinai, New York–Presbyterian, St. Luke's–Roosevelt, and many others, along with the city's public institutions, launched a wide variety of outpatient emergency services.

Counseling, of course, was a major component of the services offered. St. Vincent's Family Resource Center saw an estimated 6,000 people in the twenty-four hours following the attack. Several hundred families arrived at Cabrini seeking relatives and friends lost in the attack and were provided counseling as well. Beth Israel sent staff to ground zero to provide grief counseling to workers at the site. According to an official of the Greater New York Hospital Association, Mt. Sinai operated a twenty-four-hour hotline for two weeks, using eight phone lines to offer telephone counseling to community residents "too frightened to leave their homes." New York–Presbyterian Hospital helped a variety of "companies and organizations to provide onsite group counseling and follow-up counseling to their employees."[99] Though the DMH's LIFENET played an essential role in the weeks immediately following the attack, it was primarily a referral system and could not guarantee the quality or appropriateness of the care received.

Despite the outpouring of immediate assistance from individuals, private organizations, and public agencies, it soon became clear that planning was needed beyond the short term. Neal Cohen, a psychiatrist and New York City's commissioner of health at the time, announced just a week after the attack that it was "now time to turn to tackling the longer-term impact of this tragedy." For workers engaged in cleanup and recovery, ongoing mental health services had to be provided at ground zero as well as at other sites. Further, some mechanism for coordinating the vast range of agencies and services in the city was essential. Cohen sought to convene planning meetings with the federal Substance Abuse and Mental Health Services Administration, the New York State Office of Mental Health, the United Way, the Coalition of Voluntary Mental Health Agencies, and the Greater New York Hospital Association, among others. The DMH promised to help train mental health professionals, with a special focus on the effect of the WTC event on children.[100] "Project Liberty," the federal and state emergency program set up to fund emergency services and counseling at workplaces, schools, and homes in the metropolitan region, provided $22.7 million, with $14 million reserved for New York City itself.[101]

But as administrators and researchers alike focused on this planning, fundamental problems emerged almost immediately. It was obvious that offering even minimal short-term care was an enormous undertaking, given the area's large population and the lack of definition regarding what constituted an emergency or acute problem. An attempt to provide long-term counseling would magnify the required effort almost beyond comprehension. Some estimated that up to 10 percent of the city's population would suffer from symptoms of post-traumatic stress disorder.[102]

Barbara Aaron observes that the people working in cleanup and recovery "were facing trauma of their own in that they were doing recovery of body parts for a very, very long time in a toxic environment. A very grim job, a very dangerous job." Unlike police and firefighters, she points out, the other workers "had no preparation, no service or support network, and they were having big problems. . . . They were disconnecting from their families, because most of these people would protect their spouses and children from the experiences they had. So effectively, they kind of sealed themselves away from their families. They weren't able to provide the support or get the support. So marriages fell apart, children were in trouble, and these people moved into a different reality — they approached their job with mission and zeal." During the task itself, special ties held these workers together, but "with the ending of that experience . . . suddenly, without a whole lot of [preparation] it was over. You see the divorces, the suicides, the people who don't have jobs, they're in big trouble."

As late as June 2002, Jack Krauskopf of the 9/11 USG was concerned that although there was a system "for crisis counseling and short-term mental health assistance," it was "not clear if there is enough support for the long-term counseling and treatment needs that people who have been severely affected emotionally have." Studies estimated that up to 10 percent of New York City's 1.1 million public school students required some sort of immediate or long-term care. Aaron praised Christina Hoven, an assistant professor in the Department of Epidemiology at Columbia University's Mailman School of Public Health, for "design[ing] this unprecedented, amazing study that the Board of Education conducted on 8,300 schoolchildren across the city looking at a very broad spectrum of disorders as outcomes."

Even before the disaster, professionals had noted "a huge, unmet mental health need in the city schools throughout the New York City area."[103] But because the schools lacked sufficient money and trained staff, not even minimal counseling of students was feasible. The economic crisis overtaking the city pitted children's mental health against the need to cut spending; reductions in school budgets were already under way before September 11. Schools that sought to develop art therapy projects for traumatized children found that their art programs had been eviscerated and their staff dispersed because of cutbacks.[104]

More generally, the massive number of individuals affected and their great needs — both for short-term therapy and, in some cases, for treatment of post-traumatic stress disorder — humbled the professional world. One major problem was the limitations of public and private insurance in dealing with mental health; this failure to effectively cover services made any realistic planning for long-term psychotherapy almost impossible without a huge influx of federal and state moneys. The existing system for the delivery of extended-care services was under enormous strain. "Mental health services were already stretched to capacity before the WTC disaster," argued Patricia O'Brien, associate vice president of the Greater New York Hospital Association. "Patients were already waiting in inpatient settings because appropriate alternative levels of services were not available. . . . The development of outpatient services has been repeatedly thwarted by the state's refusal to approve new services if they will expand Medicaid costs." Even those with insurance could not expect to be completely covered for psychotherapy. O'Brien worried that "treatment for mental illnesses related to the disaster will be limited in some cases by restrictions on mental health insurance benefits."[105]

Ezra Susser, chair of the Department of Epidemiology at the Mailman School of Public Health, stresses another failing: "Thinking of it from a systems point of view, what characterized it more than anything else was fragmentation and to some degree inertia. They really weren't able to bring together the different service systems in the city, nor the research facilities. There was a lack of leadership, I would have to say." Susser believes that the New York State Office of Mental Health, "while . . . slow to respond, they did respond . . . they did try to introduce some coordination to the process. But they are not the main player here in the city. And the Department of Health was never able to exert leadership on the mental health side."[106]

By August 2002, the September 11th Fund had established policies for financing mental health services that enabled all those directly affected by the 9/11 tragedy and their families to receive long-term coverage.

Exemplifying the myriad problems encountered by those trying to coordinate services are the persistent roadblocks to gathering basic epidemiological information about the scope and degree of mental health problems affecting workers, schoolchildren, and residents in the immediate neighborhood of the World Trade Center and in the city as a whole. Susser sees the process of conducting research as "characterized by fragmentation and rivalry. There's no means for communication among the different people doing research. Not even IRBs [institutional review boards] communicate. There must be three hundred studies at least going on in the city now in mental health and research and nobody can even list them for you. They often approach the same people. It's just complete chaos." And yet, he acknowledges, "there have been some great studies done."

The long-term effect of the crisis on the provision of social services is still uncertain, but two somewhat contradictory tendencies have surfaced. On the one hand, traditional distinctions between the "worthy" and "unworthy," the "truly needy" and those "not truly in need," that have governed the distribution of welfare and charity services by government and social service agencies alike for the past two centuries were suspended — though only in the short term, reemerging as the immediate crisis passed. On the other hand, the crisis has forced the social service community to confront whether making such traditional distinctions between groups of needy or dependent people will hamper planning for future emergencies.

The Need to Protect the Public Health Infrastructure

The emerging focus on bioterrorism in public health has had the unexpected effect of reinvigorating the drive to support and strengthen the public health infrastructure in New York City and throughout the nation. Some have argued that only by buttressing their basic functions will health-related agencies be able to deal effectively with the special cases of chemical warfare, bioterrorism, or even destruction on a scale as massive as that of the World Trade Center. Andrew Goodman, New York City's associate commissioner of community health works, suggests that the efforts behind a city's health are rarely in the forefront of people's consciousness: "Every day we drink the water and assume it's safe. What people don't realize is there's an ongoing activity to ensure that that happens." It is only during a moment of crisis like the anthrax episode "that people appreciate the need for ongoing surveillance and ongoing capability around some very basic functions."

Benjamin Mojica, former deputy commissioner of health and director of the division of health, sums it up this way: Emergencies are the kinds of events that

> we in public health do not generally think of as something we have to deal with. . . . We have to rethink our mission, and find out exactly where we fit [into] all of these emergencies. We have not really thought of ourselves as responders to anything like this before, because we thought that was the Department of Environmental Protection, that's environmental conservation, that's transportation, that's law enforcement. But there's always some public health impact with this kind of disaster. There is post-traumatic stress syndrome. . . . We need to look at these things and see what kinds of ramifications they may have in the health of the public.

Although health department officials were assured in the midst of the crisis that resources would be made available for planning, there is now a real fear that the city's and state's budget crises will undercut the health infrastructure. Despite new moneys available from the federal government, units of the Department of Health were instructed to trim their budgets, and a hiring freeze was put into effect in 2002. The administrators of all divisions were informed that they would be able to replace only one of every two workers.[107] There seemed to be little immediate effect on services; for example, Lucindy Williams has seen a slight reduction in the budget of the STD clinics she manages but no substantial impact on their ability to serve their clients.[108] Nevertheless, it is not clear which force will prevail: the new awareness of the breadth of health services needed, which would logically lead to an expansion in the purview of the Department of Health or other agencies of local government, or the imperative to cut budgets in the face of local and state money woes.

The Need for City-State Coordination

Cooperation between the city and the state in response to the WTC disaster was extensive, but observers noted that in the immediate aftermath of the attack there was "intermittent confusion as to which state or local agency was 'in charge' on any given issue."[109] In contemplating changes in the legal structure for future public health emergencies, Wilfredo Lopez, general counsel of New York City's Department of Health, acknowledged that in New York both the mayor and the governor have the power to declare a state of emergency. He feared that new legislation would strengthen the state's powers at the expense of the city's and advised that "the fundamental structure of New York's existing law, which mandates to local government a primary role in emergency response, should not be altered." Indeed, in his view the ability of the city's health department to respond to health dangers quickly and efficiently is a strength of existing law: "The health officer needs to be able to act without waiting for a situation to be recognized as terrorism or to escalate to an emergency."[110]

Yet this struggle for power between city and state is occurring in the larger context of the past half century's emphasis on individualism, local control, and dependence on the private sector, which has led to a disintegration of the sense of community — and that, in turn, has undercut public health–related activities and authority. The crisis highlighted the delicate balancing act of the health agencies. On the one hand, many of them, including the Department of Health and private social welfare agencies, looked for direction from public officials, who tended to unite around a common program of returning the city to a sense of normalcy. On the other hand, the agencies had a responsibility to the public to be as accurate and honest as they could in providing information. The

Department of Health was alternately praised and condemned for trying to reconcile these two obligations in the anthrax case. But in monitoring the air in Lower Manhattan, when information was ambiguous and public perception of the potential hazard was not, the city's health agencies were less successful. Andrew Goodman says that the situation in Lower Manhattan taught the Department of Health "the need that the public has for the public health people to really be there in a very physical, consistent way, to address a lot of concerns." Similarly, the Board of Education too closely identified itself with the larger political and economic objective of returning Lower Manhattan to normal, thereby incurring the wrath of parents in the schools around the WTC.

Public Trust and Public Health

At the local level, one important theme that emerges from various discussions of the responses to 9/11 and to the anthrax incidents is the contradictory pressure exerted by officials: they urge us to return to a sense of normalcy and routine while at the same time encouraging us to maintain our vigilance and a heightened state of preparedness. In the arena of public health activities, the dual demands for normalcy and vigilance have played out in strange and sometimes conflicting ways. Most concretely and immediately, as the cases of Stuyvesant High School and Lower Manhattan illustrate, our lack of certain knowledge about environmental threats posed by exposure to the chemicals, minerals, and gases created by the explosion and collapse of the towers heightened the suspicions of policy makers, scientists, and the public toward one another. At a time when government, business leaders, and the press were urging a return to everyday activities, the smells and dusts perceptible to every New Yorker served to undermine popular trust in the statements of experts and government officials.

Perhaps the key conclusion that can be reached is that for future population health policy to be effective, those with authority must open up, not shut down, the flow of information to and their communication with the population as a whole. Policy makers and health officials now understand that maintaining public access to trustworthy information is essential. As Susan Blank of the Department of Health points out, one of the lessons she learned is "the importance of communicating with the public regularly . . . the importance of being able to say, 'We don't know. We just don't know. We're going to have to take it step by step.' I think that those are some of the major things that are going to be different."

Social Welfare and Population Health

While the city's public health department needs to buttress its traditional activities and become more open, the welfare system has found some of its basic assumptions challenged by recent events. It may ultimately find its leadership moving away from age-old principles, particularly the presumed need to distinguish between the "worthy" and "unworthy" before distributing resources to clients.

Despite the increasingly stringent requirements of federal welfare policy and the constriction of resources, local social welfare agencies saw a new and enticing model for delivering resources in the response of the social welfare community to the World Trade Center disaster. Mimi Abramovitz of Hunter College's School of Social Work describes how *New York Times* reporter Nina Bernstein portrayed the Family Assistance Center at Pier 94, which she visited shortly after the attack: she declared, "It was as if the welfare state had stumbled into paradise." Bernstein meant, according to Abramovitz, that victims had "every service anyone in that situation needed. No red tape, hardly any questions asked." It showed Abramovitz that "when we want to we can provide a good service delivery system in a way that would really meet those needs" (as America had during World War II and, earlier, during the flu epidemic of 1918).

Of course, this shift was viewed by many in the social service arena as temporary, made necessary by an emergency. "A greater willingness to help people who are victimized by trauma of this horrible kind" was not accompanied, according to Abramovitz, by a similar commitment to "help people who are victimized by daily traumas of poverty, racism, and violence." She says, "So it's disturbing to watch the outpouring of generosity — which was 'we can take care of everybody,' and this paradise welfare office, and then underneath it all, afterward, we see the old dichotomies and the old divisions reappearing." In the end, the aftermath of 9/11 intensified the problems created by federal welfare reform. Getting people "from welfare to work" depends on the existence of low-paying jobs, but such jobs were the first to disappear under the pressure of the recession and the WTC disaster. Abramovitz calls it "a triple whammy. . . . The increased demand from the World Trade Center, the increased demand from the recession, the chaos because of people losing their benefits. . . . That to me is what September 11 . . . was really about. It really intensified all those things together."

Gail Nayowith, executive director of the Citizens' Committee for

Children, one of city's most venerable child welfare advocacy organizations, is especially insightful regarding the impact of 9/11 on welfare services for children. The rhetoric of creating a cohesive, responsive, and inclusive system of welfare services that emerged in the months following the attack is coming up against the historical reality of a very fragmented and disorganized system of separate agencies, each with its own agenda. Further, the resources needed to rebuild and improve the social service infrastructure so that it can serve new clients and meet new demands seem likely to be diverted elsewhere. On the one hand, there is what Nayowith calls the "core thing" — the recovery effort and the rebuilding of Lower Manhattan. On the other hand, there is "the school system and the child care system, child welfare and juvenile justice, and the family court system over here with nothing. It's like, we have to balance our budget but we're going to have to rebuild the city. Well, how does that work?"[111] According to the September 11th Fund, the money coming in to nonprofits was primarily (49 percent) earmarked for distribution directly as cash assistance for clients. As a result, agencies were unable to hire new staff and obtain other essential infrastructure needs despite the new demand on the services. Only 13 percent of the money raised went to fund services provided by community organizations.[112]

Nayowith emphasizes the disjuncture between short-term responses and longer-term needs, which threatens to badly weaken mental health services for children and, more broadly, the mental health system as a whole. "The government responded in a way that was both impressive and alarming," Nayowith argues. "I think from a crisis perspective, [the government] really stepped up and brought people together and tried to figure it out." But "to layer a trauma crisis response on top of a pretty creaky infrastructure . . . doesn't really make for a long-term solution that's going to be good for kids and families."

Certainly, one general problem that confronted all agencies and actors after the terrorist attacks was the conflict between the desire of politicians and bureaucracies to calm a terrified population and their obligation to describe honestly and forthrightly what was and was not known. This issue becomes particularly pressing when we consider the enormous uncertainties about what environmental dangers might be associated with possible chemical, biological, or radiological attacks. One clear lesson from 9/11 is that the integrity of the agencies responsible for seeing to the population's health outweighs the dubious value of reassurances that are flimsy or are contradicted by people's everyday experience.

The city's experience in the months following the attack illustrates the difficulty of establishing responsible policies when we lack scientific knowledge about the potential health hazards of dust, debris, and toxic materials in the neighborhoods and schools near the World Trade Center site. Further, given the immediate threats the disaster posed to the population's health it is important to note the innovations both in programs and thinking that occurred right after the attacks. Particularly crucial was the swift (though temporary) shedding by (mostly) voluntary agencies in the social service and mental health sectors of long-standing social welfare practice and ideology so that they could deliver services to those in need, irrespective of social class, ability to pay, or judgments of moral worth. It is unfortunate that some of the lessons learned after September 11 were forgotten soon after the crisis had passed.

TWO

EMERGENCY PREPAREDNESS, BIOTERRORISM, AND THE STATES

The newspaper headlines were stark and eerie: "Efforts to Calm the Nation's Fears Spin Out of Control," "Local Public Health Officials Seek Help," "This Is Not a Test," "State Can't Handle Bioterrorist Attack," "Scared into Action." And the pictures that accompanied them were worse: investigators in moon suits; children ridden with smallpox; cold, stark laboratories staffed by masked personnel. State and local health departments were now supposed to be on a "war footing," as one head-line noted.[1] Health officials, knowing that their historical role was as the first line of defense against infectious disease, were simultaneously ener-gized and terrified by the prospect that their actions could be responsible for protecting or damaging the health of an entire state, or even the nation. How should they react? What were their goals? their limitations?

Public health is a methodical discipline, historically rooted in the col-lection of data, the tracking of disease outbreaks, and laboratory and epi-demiological investigation, work often done out of the public eye. But the events of September 11, 2001, and the anthrax incidents that came to light in October placed state public health agencies in the spotlight to a degree not experienced since the great epidemics of influenza, polio, and whooping cough during the first half of the twentieth century. Many officials felt overwhelmed, and the limitations of surveillance systems, laboratories, and treatment and social services became all too apparent. Almost overnight, state public health services were pulled into a cooper-ative campaign as part of the nation's defenses. As they viewed the beleaguered staff and limited laboratory space and supplies, and considered their general inexperience with bioterrorism, policy makers profoundly reevaluated — in ways sometimes naïve, sometimes quite sophisticated — the place of population health services in the country's antiterrorism and emergency preparedness systems.

Fear of terrorism, and specifically bioterrorism, thrust state agencies onto center stage in the broader arena of emergency preparedness and national security. Academics and public commentators alike argued that a new conception of traditional emergency responders was now upon us. Newspapers asserted, "Firefighters, police officers, and other first responders will be on the front lines of a terrorist attack. . . . But in a bioterrorist attack, the people on the front lines will be the practicing physicians who will diagnose and treat diseases, and public health epidemiologists and laboratory personnel who will determine who has been exposed" to a host of biological and chemical agents.[2] From established academics and public health professionals to conservative think tanks and state officials, everyone agreed that "nowadays protection from disease is nothing short of national defense."[3] State government agencies were called on to play a new and crucial role in emergency preparedness.

In his opening address to the American Public Health Association (APHA) annual meeting just a few weeks after the initial anthrax attacks, Secretary of the U.S. Department of Health and Human Services Tommy Thompson declared, "We must take this opportunity to do everything we can to strengthen the public health system."[4] Not just public health spokespeople but commentators across the political spectrum seized on the promise of federal bioterrorism money as a possible salve for the system's inadequacies; the latter also saw it as a way to buttress ideological and political goals. One fellow at the conservative American Enterprise Institute criticized public health leadership for having a "social justice agenda" that was a distraction from its true calling: "The upheaval of September 11 poses a momentous opportunity for public health to reclaim its proper focus: to protect the population from disease." Citing a 1988 Institute of Medicine study that described the public health infrastructure as being in "disarray," she argued that "that function has suffered for many years."[5] Mohammed Akhtar, executive director of the APHA, disputed this narrow construal of public health but agreed that severe weaknesses existed in the public health system that were the "result of neglect of many decades. . . . Since we conquered many infectious diseases, there have been no major outbreaks, so we continued to cut down on the system. It is at a point that it needs to be rebuilt and modernized."[6]

Those within and outside public health departments and government offices had differing views on what constituted preparedness in general and bioterrorism preparedness in particular. Local health officials, worried about the weaknesses in their agencies' programs, sometimes came into conflict with general government — state elected government officials and their staffs — who were focused on a broader array of population health needs. Those concerned with public health at the state level believed that new federal money could enable state and local agencies to rebuild, even expand, their infrastructures. They hoped that the money would be used both to prepare the nation for an emergency and to bolster general public health programs. But even in the immediate weeks after 9/11, some public health agency administrators feared that the new emphasis on bioterrorism would distort public health priorities. A narrow focus on health as an adjunct to national defense could undermine their broader mission to provide a wide range of other services.

Unlike public health officials, whose perspectives were shaped by their agencies' pressing needs, many legislators, governors, and members of their staffs concentrated on the glaring weaknesses in the social services system, on hospital care facilities, and on the broader threat of terrorism and bioterrorism alike. In addition, they were dismayed that more had not been done to strengthen emergency response coordination within and between states.

These early hopes and fears were framed by national crisis and far-reaching social, economic, and political events. The economic recession that had begun before 9/11 was greatly exacerbated as travel and consumer spending nearly halted after the terrorist attacks. Strained state finances led to budget cuts in numerous sectors, including health. As legislators moved further and further away from the events of late 2001, population health preparedness became just one of a number of different priorities jockeying for attention in tough fiscal times. In early 2002, federal grants distributed by the Centers for Disease Control and Prevention (CDC) and the Health Resources and Services Administration (HRSA) provided a substantial infusion of funds for specific health-related activities and programs intended to prepare for bioterrorism by improving the public health infrastructure. But the federal mandate in late 2002 for a major smallpox inoculation campaign dramatically changed the debate within state governments about where resources should be spent and how personnel should be allocated. In the end, the rapidly planned program was seen as a distraction both by those in general government concerned with bioterrorism preparedness and by state public health administrators.

Fiscal crises and political agendas were not the only influences on thinking about population health after 9/11. Highlighting the sometimes conflicting priorities of those in public health and those focused primarily on law enforcement and national security were the draft Emergency Health Powers Model Act (hereafter referred to as the draft Model Act); the poor federal handling — criticized by many with whom we spoke — of the anthrax episode, encapsulated in the confusing messages sent out by Tommy Thompson; and the smallpox inoculation campaign. These efforts also helped encourage a discussion of how public health agencies should respond regionally and even nationally to the threat of biological or chemical attacks.

Years after the attacks, many public health officials still perceived tremendous ambiguities in what the stress on bioterrorism and emergency preparedness meant to them. Some saw it as a call to strengthen the existing public health infrastructure or to build population health services more broadly; some saw it as narrowly concerned with smallpox, anthrax, emergency care, border protection, and the like. While all these formulations are to some degree complementary, they also created competition for scarce resources.

THE CHALLENGE OF BIOTERRORISM

Public health officials readjusted their initial expectations as the impact of 9/11 receded. At first, many believed that a new federal emphasis on bioterrorism would revitalize their field. Indeed, some serious weaknesses in the public health infrastructure were addressed. But many public health agency and government officials at the state level were wary of the stress on national defense, which they feared could result in the neglect of other programs key to improving the population's health.

Public Health: A Brief Historical Overview

September 11 helped galvanize the nation against terrorism, and the anthrax outbreaks in October 2001 and the mobilization against smallpox a few months later thrust public health and public health agencies into the national spotlight. But these episodes also stimulated influential people inside and outside government to see prevention, surveillance, and disease reporting — traditionally responsibilities of public health departments — as integral to the country's national defense system. Public health has historically played a role in national defense efforts. Malaria and yellow fever control have been crucial to American military campaigns from early-twentieth-century interventions in Latin America to World War II and Vietnam. As Robert Stroube, commissioner of the Virginia Department of Health, points out, the Epidemic Intelligence Service at the CDC had its origins in the cold war.[7]

The events of 2001 to 2003 — specifically, the threats of anthrax, smallpox, SARS (severe acute respiratory syndrome), monkeypox, and ricin — underscore the historical transformations in the field of public health. Throughout the nineteenth and early twentieth centuries, traditional preventive public health activities were essential to the growth and stability of cities and states. Rampant epidemic diseases such as cholera, smallpox, diphtheria, and influenza undermined not only the health of young and old alike but also the economic well-being of the country's growing industrial and commercial centers, including New York, Chicago, Philadelphia, and New Orleans. By undertaking quarantines, isolation, and surveillance and by providing pure water, sewerage systems, and street cleaning, public health departments became central agencies in municipal and state reform efforts. But in the twentieth century, their very success in campaigning to improve and reform housing, sanitation, and nutrition; to develop sewerage systems; to provide inoculations against infectious diseases; and to offer health programs, especially those targeting women and children, gradually led the public to view these departments as relatively unimportant.[8]

Thus, by the second decade of the twentieth century, public health officials were noting in their annual reports that longer-term illnesses were growing more prominent. By the 1920s, chronic diseases were the main cause of mortality in the United States, and many public health departments had begun programs aimed at reducing the rates of tuberculosis, heart disease, cancer, stroke, and other illnesses. As the century progressed, despite such periodic outbreaks as polio epidemics into the 1950s, the influenza pandemics of 1957 and 1968, or AIDS and multidrug-resistant tuberculosis since the 1980s, infectious diseases waned as the focus of public health activities.

Public health activities had retained their prominence and their political and cultural authority throughout the first half of the twentieth century. But the growing importance of new medical technologies and treatments for infectious disease began to overshadow traditional public health techniques. The use of antibiotic therapies for individual patients with such diseases as scarlet fever or rheumatic heart disease, for example, shifted spending priorities from public to personal health services. The vaccines developed for polio, diphtheria, measles, and mumps were public health triumphs that, ironically, further undercut the rationale for extensive public health interventions after the 1950s. The public came to envision a future in which society would be freed from infections by antibiotics and vaccines and individuals' diseases would be treated or cured by individual physicians—rather than by public health activities. Moreover, in many areas population health services for the poor were shifting away from public health departments. "As new insurance programs were developed for the indigent population (e.g., SCHIP [the State Children's Health Insurance Plan, which is part of Medicaid], Medicaid expansions)," Stroube observes, "many state and federal leaders thought the funding for public health could be cut as there would be less need for indigent care." As a result, "revenues dried up."[9] Others argue that in fact more money was available than before, though it was distributed differently. Many city and county health departments ran inadequately staffed and insufficiently funded health clinics for the poor that relied mainly on city and county moneys; Medicaid and SCHIP promised to support them, if the cities would set their payment structure to make them eligible for Medicaid matching funds. But the growth of their Medicaid programs forced some states to cut other, state-only health services to balance their budgets.

As the field's status diminished and reliance on health care institutions as the primary defense against disease grew, those concerned with the maintenance of the public health infrastructure faced a conundrum. Because public health departments were no longer perceived as central to preserving the population's health, their appeals for more funding and resources to address fissures in the existing public health system were often viewed as merely self-interested. The public and the political leadership no longer understood or sympathized with professional public health officials' goals or activities, as critical components of their original mandate were moved into departments of sanitation, environmental protection, housing, and hospitals, and as their profession became more isolated and specialized. Some lamented the resultant chronic underfunding of both public health and population health activities, but others saw public health officials as responsible for their own predicament: they had become elite professionals, defined their mandate too narrowly, and isolated themselves from more general concerns of population health.[10]

Bioterrorism:
"Where Bad Bugs and Bad Guys Come Together"

The federal promises of money in late 2001 and early 2002 raised expectations that what many considered to be the long neglect of state and local public health agencies had finally come to an end. Those in state public health agencies viewed the events of late 2001 as potentially empowering, reversing what they perceived to be their century-long decline in status and authority. "Before, they left public health out [at the state level]," says Anne Harnish, assistant director of the Ohio Department of Health. "But bioterrorism brought us to the table and showed that we do have expertise."[11] Similarly, Ronald Cates, chief operating officer of the Missouri Department of Health and Senior Services, voices the position of many public health officials: "A lot of people who couldn't spell 'public health' now saw public health as the equivalent of the Department of Defense."[12] Even in Massachusetts, a state with the oldest department of health in the country, administrators and politicians believe that "public health was never really an equal partner at the table . . . in the past" — that is, in the past half century — but "became an equal partner as it was called upon to safeguard our water supply," protect the airports, and prevent the importation of biological agents into the state.[13]

Some state officials not directly involved in public health had a somewhat different perception of its place in history and in emergency preparedness. Massachusetts State Senator Harriette Chandler believes that the discussion of anthrax fundamentally transformed how state officials view public health. "The anthrax scare that we had was more than a public safety scare," she recalls. "It required public health, it required testing, and it required knowledgeable people. But it also required the two groups [public safety and public health] to work together and to understand where the FBI comes in, local and state police, and if there's a role for municipal authorities. In that paradigm public health was basically the quarterback. We've never had that before." Chandler sees the need for a public health response as part of a broader problem: "It also showed all of the weaknesses that we have in terms of a national disaster or emergency."

Even in states whose government agencies were vigilant in carrying out emergency planning for natural disasters, administrators in departments of health saw the anthrax episode as a watershed. Angela Coron, associate director of the Department of Health Services in California — a state accustomed to planning for and coping with earthquakes, fires, floods, and drought — remembers that "we took advantage of bioterrorism funds for California and Los Angeles to expand our capacity to respond statewide." California, like many states, has a decentralized system with sixty-one jurisdictions for public health, which came to be "included in emergency preparedness more and more," because anthrax and smallpox are "where bad bugs and bad guys come together."[14]

Across the country, administrators saw bioterrorism as an enormous opportunity to effect a sea change in public attitudes. They hoped that the money could be used both to prepare the nation and to support general public health programs. Dennis Perrotta, then state epidemiologist for the Texas Department of Health (now associate professor of epidemiology and biosecurity at the University of Texas School of Public Health's Center for Biosecurity and Public Health Preparedness), speaks for the public health community when he observes that in disasters public health traditionally was positioned "always in the back helping. In bioterrorism, we moved to the driver's seat of the bus. . . . We have been brought to the front table. Sometimes in the past we have been well received, and sometimes not well received, but now the other players are our best friends."[15] In Arizona, Catherine Eden, once a state legislator but at the time director of the state's Department of Health Services, and David Engelthaler, then chief of the State Office of Bioterrorism and Epidemic Preparedness and Response and now state epidemiologist for the Arizona Department of Health Services, thought it was "interesting [that] the military, police, and fire . . . now know they very much need us." But it is "very new for public health to be so far out in the forefront," and the shift did not occur without a major effort by public health officials. They explain, "We had to insert ourselves into the emergency management/response community, and there has been a major culture shift in emergency management, perhaps across the country but definitely in Arizona. . . . We were able to get an understanding of the emergency management/response community and give them an understanding of us."[16]

Eden, perhaps because her background is in politics rather than public health, could see the profound change in the culture of the department as public health personnel gained "respect with the legislature and the press." State legislators paid closer attention to the possible role of departments of health in antiterrorist planning. Similarly, Mary Kramer, then president of the Iowa State Senate and subsequently a U.S. ambassador, recalls that the anthrax scare persuaded legislators to "includ[e] public health people for the first time in our emergency planning efforts."[17] In Missouri, Ronald Cates believes that in fact "public health is the lead agency." Throughout the nation, the events of 2001 led those in public health to reevaluate the accuracy of their half-century-old self-image as an underfunded and unappreciated stepchild of government.

For the first time in many years, state and local departments of health were engaging in long-term planning that could provide services that would protect against bioterrorist emergencies as well as promote population health in their states. Emergency preparedness could result in fundamental reform of public health practice. To Rice Leach, commissioner of the Kentucky Department for Public Health, it appeared that public health was recovering its old, lost focus: "This [was] the first time since polio in the 1940s and 1950s that public health has had the opportunity to shine. It's a hell of a situation, but it gives us an opportunity to strut our stuff."[18] As he told a reporter in 2002, public health has "dealt with these things in the past. . . . But since polio and tuberculosis have declined, we've not had to handle things that affected the entire system."[19] Whatever loss of prestige the field had suffered was forgotten, now that its special skills and methodologies were highly relevant.

The perceived "decline" of state and local standing in the second half of the twentieth century had been paralleled by the growing importance of new federal initiatives to address disease in general and infectious diseases more specifically. The most important was the creation within the United States Public Health Service in 1946 of the Communicable Disease Center (renamed the Center for Disease Control in 1970, the Centers for Disease Control in 1980, and the Centers for Disease Control and Prevention in 1992). This federal agency became the nexus of epidemiology, laboratory science, health surveys, and disease surveillance and reporting. Anthony Moulton, co-director of its Public Health Law Program, points out that the CDC built on state and local department strengths. Public health agencies routinely are engaged in "monitoring health of communities, including the surveillance for infectious disease . . . and monitoring unusual cases and patterns of disease and injury." The CDC also relies on close coordination with medical and public health professionals, such as private doctors, and emergency room nurses and physicians, who are often the first to notice unusual diseases or disease patterns. "One or more observant people see something amiss and may initiate quarantine [or isolation] and notify state/local public health agencies, which in turn would notify the CDC." Some very traditional public health approaches used by various states during natural dis-

asters "applied equally to biological, chemical, and radiological threats."
Once possible disease outbreaks are identified, public health laboratories
go to work and actions are taken to limit the impact of the disease on the
population: primarily inspection, isolation (the segregation of those with
symptoms), and quarantine (the segregation of those not symptomatic
but possibly exposed). Finally, Moulton notes, public health authorities
ideally do a "postmortem of the whole operation — seeing what went
right and wrong — and planning for training courses" and improvements
in infrastructure that they identify as necessary.[20] Leach summarizes these
traditional mechanisms: "In any emergency preparedness you have to
detect, identify, intercept, neutralize, and recover. In public health we do
surveillance for detection, we use labs and epidemiology for identification, we use vaccines, antibiotics, and quarantine to neutralize, and we
are the only ones who can certify that we have recovered from a problem, whether it be bioterrorism or meningitis."

The public health and emergency response communities had not been
caught completely unawares by the September 11 attacks and the
anthrax episodes. The federal government had already engaged in a number of exercises aimed at assessing the nation's preparedness for bioterrorist and chemical attacks, two of which were especially relevant for
public health officials. In May 2000 the federal government organized
mock attacks on three cities, one chemical (in Portsmouth, New
Hampshire), one radiological (in the area of Washington, D.C.), and one
involving bioweapons (in Denver). Called TOPOFF because top officials
of the U.S. government were involved, the exercise had, in the words of
observers, "illuminated problematic areas of leadership and decision
making; the difficulties of prioritization and distribution of scarce
resources; the crisis that contagious epidemics would cause in health care
facilities; and the critical need to formulate sound principles of disease
containment."[21] Also, according to Nebraska's chief medical officer, in
1999 the federal government had "made grants available in five focus
areas for bioterrorism preparedness."[22]

Not insignificantly, national concerns about the possibility of a computer system meltdown at the turn of the new century, commonly
referred to as "the Y2K bug," had also forced some state agencies to
address emergency preparedness planning. This effort revealed a great
deal about the absence of coordination within the government and
between the government and health care organizations. In June 2001 the
nonprofit Center for Strategic and International Studies, the Johns
Hopkins Center for Civilian Biodefense Studies, the ANSER Institute for

Homeland Security, and the Oklahoma National Memorial Institute for the Prevention of Terrorism put together what they called "a senior-level war game examining the national security, intergovernmental, and information challenges of a [smallpox] attack on the American homeland." This exercise, named Dark Winter, spanned thirteen days; its results suggested that inadequate planning and coordination at the state and federal levels had left the nation far from ready to confront a bioterrorist attack.[23]

As a result of these and other efforts, some states had begun to seriously plan for the possibility of massive disruptions before 9/11. For example, Norma Gyle, a former legislator and now deputy commissioner of the Connecticut Department of Public Health, notes that her state was "very fortunate," for it had been preparing studies during the two years preceding the terrorist attacks. Concerned that massive computer failures and disruptions were a real possibility on January 1, 2000, the state had "organized a command center that stood [Connecticut] in good stead." Because there was at least "one general convinced that there would be no milk left on the shelves," officials were "well organized."[24] California was also in relatively good shape, despite low morale due to the state's ongoing budget crises. Its well-developed emergency response program stayed effective because of repeated practice in dealing with natural disasters, from earthquakes and mudslides to brushfires and chemical spills. Philip Lee, who served as assistant secretary of health in both the Johnson and Clinton administrations and now teaches at the University of California at San Francisco's Institute for Health Policy Studies, said that "overall, California is better off than most states in bioterrorism preparedness. Historically, it has had a strong system of public health laboratories. . . . Chemical spills have honed the skills of hazardous materials containment teams — skills that translate well in the handling of both biological and chemical warfare attacks."[25] And labs in Colorado and Nebraska were identified as being better than those of most other states. In addition, according to the *Denver Post,* the Colorado "Department of Public Health and Environment has discovered ways to more rapidly test for such things as anthrax and plague."[26]

Such planning did not cease when the predicted disasters did not occur. Before September 11, the Connecticut Department of Public Health, like those in forty-three other states, had received a Health Alert Network grant from the CDC to improve its electronic communications systems.[27] The *Hartford Courant* reported in 2002 that the department had "made communications a major early priority . . . [and launched] a

Web site that linked health care professionals and public safety officials with the health department." This would, in the words of Warren Wollschlager, chief of staff for the Department of Public Health, "provide nearly instant information on critical resources, such as available medicines and empty hospital beds"; as a result, the "state is much better prepared to deal with a germ attack today than it was a year ago."[28]

Lack of Preparedness

Though some state departments of health had at least begun to plan for disasters, as described above, most were grossly unprepared for the terrorist attacks and their aftermath. Georges Benjamin, then director of the Maryland Department of Health and also president of the Association of State and Territorial Health Officials (ASTHO), noted in October 2001, just weeks after the planes struck the World Trade Center and the Pentagon, that "in a field where communication can save a life, some state health departments" did not have effective e-mail links with their local and county departments.[29] The *Atlanta Journal and Constitution,* citing Benjamin, reported that "public health officials have been warning for years that the [public health] system is antiquated."[30] Lack of financial support was as much to blame as failures in planning. "Public health funding has been woefully inadequate and it needs a boost," Benjamin complained, adding that the basic infrastructure of public health needed to be "enhanced . . . at local levels to fund disease-surveillance systems, to do basic medical detective work, to coordinate with local officials, hospitals, and labs."[31] The National Association of County and City Health Officials (NACCHO), in its study "Local Public Health Agency Infrastructure: A Chartbook" and elsewhere, pointed out that "most public health departments are not accessible 24 hours a day; 10 percent of the 3,000 local health departments don't have e-mail, let alone a computer network that links to hospitals and other health departments that would allow information about suspicious events to be distributed quickly."[32]

Benjamin, now the executive director of the American Public Health Association, observes, "September 11 brought home the fact that we had to do something about public health preparedness. Before, there was a small cadre of people concerned about bioterrorism and a small amount of money from the CDC on bioterrorism that was a specialty program and not well funded." And those people were not listened to but "were seen as doomsayers. The West Nile virus episode [first detected in North America in 1999] put people into a response mode, at least on the East Coast. They became tuned in to interagency cooperation to respond to an environmental event. Anthrax rolled out very slowly, insidiously. We knew it was about to come but hoped that it wouldn't . . . and then [were] shocked that it happened, but still there was an avoidance of its implications." After some days of confusion, there was "a quick response and great concern about the impact."[33]

Benjamin's summary reflects the growing worries about the public health infrastructure that preceded the attacks. A CDC report published only months before 9/11 detailed the terrible state of most county and city public health departments across the country. Of the 3,000 surveyed, approximately 78 percent were directed by people with no graduate training. The CDC found that "only one-third of the U.S. population [was] effectively served by public health agencies." Even the most mundane technologies were lacking in many health departments around the country: "In a test of e-mail capacity, only 35 percent of messages to local health departments were delivered successfully."[34] The CDC lamented that "the U.S. public health infrastructure, which protects the nation against the spread of disease and environmental and occupational hazards, is still structurally weak in nearly every area." In summary, the CDC found that "our local public health agencies lack basic equipment. . . . Our public health laboratories are old and unsafe. . . . Our public health physicians and nurses are untrained in new threats like West Nile virus and weaponized microorganisms."[35]

In the two years following the 9/11 attacks, state departments of health throughout the country sought to determine their own state of preparedness and to define exactly what *preparedness* meant. According to Southern California's *North County Times,* one nationwide survey found "90 percent of county governments . . . unprepared for biological or chemical attacks." Tom Milne, former executive director of NACCHO, observed that "a significant number of local health departments have no high speed access to the Internet, no way of sharing data." In fact, Illinois doctors reporting outbreaks have to contact the state by telephone or mail — a process described by John Lumpkin, formerly the state's public health chief, as "basically 1920s technology for monitoring disease."[36] In Illinois, reported the *Chicago Tribune* in November 2001, the state's three labs — in Chicago, Springfield, and Carbondale — were not linked electronically. The health department acknowledged that the latter two "labs also need to be upgraded so they can perform more sophisticated tests on site. . . . And new equipment that can deliver results of biological tests in one hour, as opposed to 48 hours under conventional testing methods, is needed." Iowa was in a similar position, according to Mary Gilchrist, then president of the Association of Public Health Laboratories and director of the University of Iowa's Hygienic Laboratory, who added, "Our personnel are very limited."[37]

To help remedy the flaws in the public health infrastructure thrown into relief by the anthrax attack, the $2.9 billion bioterrorism appropriations bill signed by President George W. Bush on January 10, 2002, included $1.1 billion for the states, territories, and three cities — Chicago, Los Angeles, and New York — so that they might "develop comprehensive bioterrorism preparedness plans, upgrade infectious-disease surveillance and investigation, enhance the readiness of hospital systems to deal with large numbers of casualties, expand public health laboratory and communications capacities, and improve connectivity between hospitals and city, local, and state health departments to enhance disease reporting."[38] The moneys were divided into three components. All the states were given up front 20 percent of their per capita allotment — in most cases several million dollars — so that they might develop plans for using the remainder, which was made available after the plans were reviewed. The bulk of it consisted of grants from the CDC specifically "targeted to supporting bioterrorism, infectious diseases, and public health emergency preparedness activities." Finally, the Health Resources and Services Administration provided funding to "be used by states to create regional hospital plans to respond in the event of a bioterrorism attack."[39] To get the money, the governor's office, often relying on the state department of health, submitted bioterror preparedness plans to the Department of Health and Human Services; requirements included hiring "at least one epidemiologist . . . for each metropolitan area with a population greater than 500,000" and "develop[ing] a communications system that provides a 24/7 flow of health information among hospital, state, and local health officials and law enforcement."[40] In addition, the CDC targeted "preparedness planning and readiness assessment, surveillance and epidemiology capacity, laboratory capacity, Health Alert Network/communications, risk communication and health information dissemination, and education and training."[41]

To some extent, the expectations of officials at the federal and the state levels never matched. State officials viewed the billions of dollars pledged by the federal government as their means of saving a public health infrastructure badly damaged by long neglect. But those in the federal government saw the money made available through the CDC and HRSA as a small part of the war on terrorism — funds that promised only modest benefits to the infrastructure. In some states, some small improvement did come about. For example, in Virginia, according to Robert Stroube, the renewed attention to public health and the relationships fostered by the governor's office were "beneficial to the public health system." Because they had the "opportunity to actually interface with the governor's office," public health workers had "unprecedented visibility: The governor provided additional state funds for public health preparedness because he thought preparedness was as much a state responsibility as a federal one. Additionally, the governor authorized the state health department to hire an additional 140–150 people in full-time positions to carry out these new responsibilities."[42]

Many states wrestled with the necessity of hiring trained personnel. Georges Benjamin said that officials in Maryland were "trying to invest to get an adequate workforce. The good news is states have the money to do it, but the bad news is there [are] not a lot of people with those qualifications," and "there may not be enough qualified people to fill the jobs." Maryland, he noted, was "hiring in all areas — epidemiology, laboratories, public relations, and information technology," and the state was "hopeful with two (local) public health schools that we'll find the staff we need." Dennis Perrotta pointed out that Texas would hire fifty more public health workers at the state level alone, helping to staff four new laboratories, provide information to the public, and plan on the regional level to prevent bioterrorism.[43] Washington State, a geographically large and politically and socially diverse state with only one school of public health, found itself in a more difficult position. Secretary of Health Mary Selecky believed that finding qualified personnel would not be easy: "You don't create epidemiologists overnight."[44] In Kansas, particularly in the western counties, health departments and hospitals were being seriously undermined as part of a larger problem: depopulation. Melvin Neufeld, a member of the Joint Legislative Budget Committee of the Kansas House of Representatives, describes local battles over attempts to consolidate school districts and other governmental programs in counties that feel that their independence and integrity are at risk. Further, there were few trained health professionals willing to move to Kansas, a state whose major industries — agriculture and aerospace — have been in decline.[45] Other states, such as Nebraska and Illinois, succeeded in using the grants to coordinate health services across county lines. But recruiting qualified personnel clearly remains extremely difficult. In 2005 the Council of State and Territorial Epidemiologists examined the training of the epidemiologists across the country who were "working on terrorism preparedness programs"; 26 percent (108) out of a total of 424 had bachelor's degrees and 6 percent (25) had only associate's degrees or high school diplomas. Twenty percent had no formal training or academic course work in epidemiology.[46]

Dual Use for Bioterrorism Funding

Years before the anthrax mailings made bioterrorism a household word, some experts were suggesting that there was no contradiction between improving the overall public health infrastructure and ensuring that the nation could protect itself from bioterrorist attacks. In 1999, in a prescient article describing the government's growing attention to bioterrorism as a real threat, Sydney Freedberg and Marilyn Serafini quoted the terrorism expert Richard Falkenrath, then at Harvard's Kennedy School of Government, on the benefits of bioterrorism money as a salve for the problems plaguing state departments of health: "Even in the crucial area where existing assets are inadequate — public health — filling the gaps has benefits far beyond biowar. New multipurpose drugs, new vaccines, and above all, a revived public health surveillance system are all independently desirable because they help you get a handle on naturally occurring diseases which are in all respects more common and more damaging to American citizens." Other experts quoted in the article agreed. James M. Hughes, director of the National Center for Infectious Diseases at CDC, declared: "This money is going to be well-spent, strengthening national, state and local capacity to deal with infectious agents, even if a biological attack does not occur. . . . To stop both biowar and natural disease outbreaks, the steps you have to take are the same." Surgeon General David Satcher saw these bioterrorism funds as a way to counter what he described as "decades of decay and neglect to the public health system." Fortunately or unfortunately, "bioterrorism has really gotten the attention of people, [when] perhaps we've had trouble getting their attention before."[47]

In the immediate aftermath of the anthrax episode, these hopes for the dual benefits of bioterrorism funding were revived. Mary Selecky, among many others, wondered if the money was going to be there for the long term, and whether it would support the public health infrastructure generally and not just address one current pressing issue. "We have had numerous communicable diseases many times before we had anthrax last fall, and we're using the same systems," she pointed out; what was needed was "a sustained, long-term investment, so . . . if headlines seem to reduce, we don't drop our attention."[48] Others similarly mixed hope and skepticism. Officials in Chicago, for example, hoped that federal funds would go "beyond hazardous-materials suits and stockpiles of penicillin to computer networks, personnel training, modern laboratories, and updated equipment that is critical in times of crisis and in routine work." Patrick Lenihan, the deputy commissioner of the Chicago Department of Public Health, told a reporter, "The day-to-day stuff that is taken for granted is just what is called upon in a threat of bioterrorism," pointing out that epidemiology and surveillance were essential to the tracking of syphilis and tuberculosis no less than anthrax and smallpox.[49]

Some state administrators see the efforts around bioterrorism as having had lasting positive effects on the public health infrastructure in their states. The Connecticut Department of Public Health's strategy "was the establishment of two hospital-based Centers of Excellence for Bioterrorism Preparedness and Response," one at Hartford Hospital and the other at Yale–New Haven Hospital. It is taking what it describes as "a leadership role in regional coordination, education, clinical care, and research to improve Connecticut's ability to respond to a large-scale bioterrorism event."[50] California had a CDC grant before September 11 for emergency planning, but in the words of Angela Coron, "September 11 focused our attention in a different way. It became very real. You look at things differently when they come home."

In Ohio, the federal government provided nearly $35 million to fund bioterrorism-related activities — $30 million from the CDC and the rest from HRSA.[51] Out of these grants, local health departments gained $11 million.[52] Anne Harnish, assistant director of the Ohio Department of Health, recalls that 9/11 forced the department to "revamp the way we looked at everything. . . . In our strategic plan we added the goal of preparedness." The department improved the relationship between "local hospitals and local health departments" and "established 24/7 communication with local health groups so all public health has benefited." She notes that bioterrorism money was critical to maintaining staffing levels: "When people were laid off, it was sometimes possible to rehire them under the bioterrorism rubric." The new focus on bioterrorism also motivated the state to reorganize its training program. The Department of Health trained 250 local health agency leaders and 413 of its own staff in the principles of their new Incident Command System, a cornerstone of managing the state's smallpox vaccination program. Hospital personnel were taught to recognize "an unusual infectious disease outbreak due to the release of a BT [bioterrorism] agent."[53] This instruction sensitized hospital staff to the importance of reporting infectious diseases to state health authorities, a legal requirement that previously had often been ignored in practice.

Virginia, home of the Pentagon and therefore a direct victim of the September 11 attacks, received more than $27 million in federal funding, all but about $3 million from the CDC. It reported using the money to hire epidemiologists and provide health planning for the thirty-five local health districts and five regions and to "implement plans for the National Pharmaceutical Stockpile and the smallpox vaccination program." The state also developed "biosafety level 3+ labs [i.e., laboratories capable of handling dangerous but not the most highly infectious agents] and a network of 90 local labs as well as 18 scientific staff to enhance biologic and chemical agent identification." Regional planning for the hospital infrastructure and disaster planning and surveillance activities were all improved as well.[54]

Lisa Kaplowitz, former director of the HIV/AIDS Center of Virginia Commonwealth University, was hired with this new federal funding as deputy commissioner for bioterrorism preparedness and response in the Virginia Department of Health (VDH); however, she soon found that her role had expanded to "emergency preparedness — an all-hazards approach." According to one report, the "health department [was now] involved in many types of disasters, natural and manmade."[55] Kaplowitz believes that the department was making good use of the funding to hire "public health response staff. About one-third of the 138 new positions have been filled, and most are expected to be filled by early next year." She adds, "A key component of our preparedness efforts is to build public health infrastructure. People must be in place, trained, and equipped with a well-planned and tested system to effectively detect and respond to any public health emergency."[56] By 2002 the VDH had hired "all key central office Emergency Preparedness and Response Staff, . . . [including] 20 of 35 district epidemiologists . . . [and] 11 of the 35 district emergency coordinators. . . . VDH's Health Alert Network has been established to ensure effective communication connectivity among public health departments, health care organizations, and other public health partners."[57] Kaplowitz recalls that though the "Health Department was very pleased with the rapid funding," there was "a lot of anger and frustration" among police and fire officials "that they were not getting the money [$3.5 billion] that was promised. . . . People were counting on it, and the legislation was never passed" until mid-2003, when the amount allocated was far less than had been expected.

Some of the least populated and most rural states — such as North Dakota, which had experienced massive flooding and other environmental disasters in the 1990s — found that the money earmarked for bioterrorism was a benefit to the state's public health infrastructure. Sheila Peterson, director of the North Dakota Office of Management and Budget's Fiscal Management Division, noted that the money helped the state to hire epidemiologists and to acquire more equipment for their labs. She does not believe that the new emphasis on bioterrorism created "a drain in resources." To the contrary, "federal moneys have enhanced our abilities so much."[58] Arvy Smith, deputy state health officer, and Brenda Vossler, bioterrorism hospital coordinator for the North Dakota Department of Health, explain that the $6.9 million that the state received from the federal government has helped them develop new capabilities in bioterrorist response. The department expected that there would be thirteen new hires. Whereas "previously [the department] had only one epidemiologist in each of six regional offices, [it] now [has] added two more. . . . Our labs needed updating and federal funding was important. . . . Our communications with partners improved dramatically. We are working on our Health Alert Network to connect emergency responders and health care providers electronically as well as improving training and coordination of public health programs throughout the state." The infusion of federal funds was of critical importance because "State budgets are very tight now. Without federal money, improvements to public health infrastructure are not possible."[59]

In the days following the anthrax episode, bioterrorism became the "top priority" for the Arizona Department of Health as well as for the entire state, according to Catherine Eden. The department had organized an emergency response system six months prior, a plan that relied "heavily on our county health department partners." But following September 11 and the anthrax mailings, the state health department took on greater responsibility for the laboratory testing of suspected anthrax cases, hoaxes, and other potential bioterrorist emergencies. Despite these added burdens, Eden and David Engelthaler recall that "we were able to cover all of our needs. . . . I don't know of any specific issue that suffered."

Kentucky received $16 million, of which $14 million came from the CDC for bioterrorism but which also aided the state in developing its public health infrastructure. The state used this money to improve its public health laboratories, upgrade coordination among various institutions, and strengthen its epidemiological and surveillance systems. Kentucky had been the site of the first test of the National Pharmaceutical Stockpile, a program begun in 1999 to ensure quick delivery of medical materiel to states and communities in the event of an emergency.[60] Rice Leach, commissioner of the Department for Public Health, remembers that "October 8 [in 2001] was the exact date that everything changed. In the middle of a meeting a person came in and said that they had a possible anthrax [attack] in three of our clinics." Within half a day, "environmental protection, police, National Guard, and other agencies came together to come up with a way to handle all the specimens." Although the state and the department "were caught somewhat flatfooted" by the anthrax scare, the "department, especially the laboratory side, worked almost around the clock to test samples," and the state had to absorb the enormous costs. "We definitely changed priorities. We had to stop doing some things. We got no new money until the CDC grant [$15 million]. We had to absorb the new planning with hospitals, med[ical] societies, etc. It was a public health emergency, and we responded."

Leach acknowledges that "the focus on bioterrorism has taken energy away from the routine monitoring that we engage in," but he also points out that it has spurred improvement of the state's communication system; now every health department in the state is in constant contact. He believes that "increasingly, people are working together better. People used to talk *about* each other and are now talking *with* each other." In his view, the states were helped immeasurably by the flexibility of the CDC under Jeff Koplan, who told them that they could "use . . . other grant money to take care of anthrax. You didn't have to dot every *i* in the grants to prove you were using it for the purpose you stated. . . . The [secretary] of health and human services is trying to make it right. I give him an A for effort." Leach even believes that the essential issue was not the lack of resources provided by the CDC: "If you had given us more than $15 million, we might not have been able to spend it effectively."

As part of Kentucky's grant from HRSA, the state was able to upgrade two animal laboratories. Leach explained to a reporter why animal labs were necessary: "The critters could be a source of terrorism" by those deliberately infecting "our milk, eggs, chickens," and seeking through them "maybe, or maybe not," to infect humans.[61] Bioterrorism provided the rationale to improve a service essential to this rural state. In Missouri as well, state officials saw the federal government as a "great partner" in the months immediately after September 11. As Ronald Cates puts it, the money was "tremendous for Missouri and helped to build a great system for the state." In Colorado, federal bioterrorism money was used to improve the public health system, whose infrastructure, according to Chuck Stout, the director of the Boulder County Health Department, "was very, very fragile." The *Denver Post* also reported that the money would be used "to hire 14 epidemiologists to help improve disease tracking" and "to improve communication among local health departments," as well as to "beef up laboratories at state facilities in Colorado Springs, Denver, Durango, Grand Junction, Greeley, and Pueblo."[62]

Mixed Reactions to Bioterrorism Funding

Though many state administrators and legislators enthusiastically supported Washington's efforts to combat bioterrorism, officials in other states, including Kansas, Louisiana, New Jersey, and Texas, had mixed reactions to the impact of federal funding on their state health departments. Perhaps J. Thomas Schedler, chair of the Health and Welfare Committee of the Louisiana State Senate, put it most succinctly: "I guess there's always a good news/bad news scenario in everything you do. I think the good news from a public health standpoint is that the area of public health in Louisiana probably needed some drastic overhauls and new influx of money for years and years, and sometimes it takes a crisis to make that happen."[63]

Specifically, according to Schedler, Louisiana "for a long time needed to upgrade [its] lab facilities. . . . That is occurring in several sections of the state [where it] would probably not have occurred without this crisis. . . . Communication lines between hospitals and the Department of Health and Hospitals have been improved. [We stockpiled] certain types of drugs that were not there before, and even though we had limited supplies, it certainly put a focus on those types of things." The other areas that benefited were "looking at things on a regional basis . . . and the structure of command in the event of a biological attack or some other crisis. . . . So that's the good side of it." But, Schedler points out, "there's a down side as well." The new emphasis on emergency preparedness "has put an untold strain on our budget. . . . The states are having severe trouble right now with Medicaid and budgets and downturns of sales tax, corporate taxes, and the like. So the timing of this couldn't have come at a worse time, but nonetheless, we have seen a tremendous shift into that arena."

In New Jersey, George DiFerdinando, Jr., deputy commissioner of the state's Department of Health and Senior Services, notes that because the state was directly affected by anthrax cases at the Camden Post Office and was also immediately across the river from the World Trade Center disaster, it was especially hard hit by anxiety in the weeks following 9/11. "At that time," DiFerdinando recalls, "I was functioning in an operational role [as acting commissioner], and on 9/11, though we were not the lead agency in New Jersey, we could sign executive orders to let people get the medical records of missing relatives and to allow for the release of names of missing people." He remembers that they received "an agreement from Tommy Thompson from Health and Human Services that state agencies could use funds from other programs, for example, tuberculosis, for emergency purposes." While the state could therefore "reallocate people as needed," the strains on the system were enormous. "If there had been another explosion in Philly, then it would have been very difficult to decide where to put resources." Federal money, he adds, was especially important for "improving public health and health care infrastructure."[64]

In "Lessons from the Anthrax Attacks of 2001: The New Jersey Experience," Eddy Bresnitz, the state epidemiologist, and George DiFerdinando succinctly describe the crisis that had faced the state: "New Jersey became the focal point of the bioterrorism-related anthrax outbreak in the United States. At least four letters containing weapons-grade anthrax spores passed through the Trenton Postal Processing and Distribution Center [PDC] in Hamilton Township, New Jersey, in September and October 2001. The spore-filled letters caused widespread contamination." In all, 1,100 workers were exposed, and five of them contracted anthrax; one New Jerseyan who did not work in the post office also became ill with anthrax. The state immediately established a surveillance system that included sixty-one area hospitals in fifteen counties. This effort created tremendous strains on the hospital staff and taught the state that "in the absence of a credible exposure or apparent outbreak, the most critical function is to have a sound surveillance infrastructure for routinely notifiable conditions, such as the more common infectious diseases that must be reported by law. This infrastructure establishes the relationships, lines of communication, and awareness of reporting procedures that are critical to identifying index cases and monitoring for other cases in the event of an intentional exposure. Most outbreaks are not detected by surveillance systems but by clinicians who suspect an unusual event and notify public health officials."[65]

Bresnitz and DiFerdinando learned that in many ways, "the response to the contamination of the Trenton PDC was fundamentally the response to a typical airborne contamination of a workplace." But the one major difference was that "the Trenton PDC exposure . . . occurred within a regional and national context of a national state of emergency, and the situation gained resonance beyond any typical workplace safety issue. As a crime scene and as part of an emerging national war on terrorism, the contamination of the Trenton PDC and the public health response involved all levels of the U.S. government and all forms of media."[66] For that reason, DiFerdinando stresses, federal money coming into the state following 9/11 "went for public health and health care infrastructure."

Though New Jersey's experience with federally allocated bioterrorism money was generally good, and though it was given unusual leeway in allocating its resources, the state still experienced difficulties. The first major problem was in planning for services when the federal budget itself was in disarray and decisions about funding occurred "only five months before the start of the fiscal year." The state did not know what cuts might occur in existing programs, whether it would be able to balance those cuts with new money, or whether federal mandates would dictate how the money should be spent. The second problem was that the emphasis on emergency preparedness distorted some priorities. DiFerdinando explains, "Before September 11, New Jersey had a substance abuse task force" that estimated that "there might be a million people in need of treatment," of whom 80,000 at any time might voluntarily ask for treatment. "In August of 2001 we had high hopes for extra dollars" to treat 40,000 people. "But no one heard that after 9/11. How could it be any other way after money started flowing for bioterrorism?" DiFerdinando and the state had expected increased revenues from the cigarette tax, which had recently been raised to $1.50 per pack. "This would have allowed the $30 million commitment for tobacco control to rise to $45 million. But with the budget constraints, the governor is now proposing $10 million." The increase in revenues that the health department had expected would now be diverted to other state needs. In the end, DiFerdinando believes the problems facing New Jersey were caused by · "a confluence of the state budget crisis, bioterrorism, and smallpox."

Texas: A Case Study of the Mixed Blessings of Bioterrorism Money

Texas, a huge state with 254 counties and a highly decentralized county-based public health system, was nearly overwhelmed by the anthrax episode. Jack Colley, state coordinator in the Division of Emergency Management of the Texas Department of Public Safety, recalls that "with anthrax we quit trying to keep track of the number of undetermined white powders. What did we learn? Before we had eight labs working from 8 to 5, and now we have ten labs with 24/7 capacity." The state quickly became skilled at "how to process, detect, and give feedback, that is, confirm or deny, quicker." It "treated every single reported white powder as potential anthrax" and mobilized to swiftly "detect biological, chemical, and radiological agents."[67]

The problems facing a state the size and complexity of Texas, with both major cities and distant rural counties, were daunting. An article by the Texas Association of Counties reported that emergency medical services and fire department personnel wanted new equipment, and county officials wanted to ensure that localities have "plans in place to handle a biological outbreak and have the capabilities to detect, treat, and contain a biological incident. Local hospitals and health departments in the county need to be able to recognize signs of illness, report the suspect diseases, treat mass casualties, and provide necessary antibiotics or vaccines." The article concluded that "since Sept. 11, the Texas Department of Health has been gearing up preparation and response activities, but the state system relies on local public health entities to identify attacks, and little is known about levels of readiness at the local level, especially in rural areas." It found a number of problems with the state's emergency response systems, including poor infectious disease surveillance programs at the local level and "many health care professionals" without "the capability to handle bioterrorism." Localities, like the state, were unable to cope with the increased demands placed on them at the very time when budgets were contracting and tax revenues were falling. The representatives of many agencies told the state of their concerns about the cost of security, and many counties sought additional funding from the state and the federal government.[68]

Governor Rick Perry "authorized the use of more than $6 million from the health department's budget for improving bioterrorism preparedness, including adding staff, upgrading laboratory equipment, and improving training." In addition, reported the Associated Press, the state received $2.1 million from the Department of Mental Health and Mental Retardation to address post-traumatic stress. The health department, according to Dennis Perrotta, also began "working with other agencies to improve communication systems, prepare health facilities, and create a plan for getting medicines and improving detection of outbreaks."

Perhaps what came through most forcefully was that "a strong and flexible public health system is the best defense."[69]

Perrotta, who had served as a consultant to the Asthma Surveillance Case Definition Work Group of the Association of State and Territorial Health Officials, had a broad view of the crisis affecting state health departments across the nation. He became acutely aware both of the tremendous support given to the states by federal bioterrorism money and of the attendant problems. The CDC grants were welcomed, but the "big surprise was the amount of work that the CDC and HHS [the Department of Health and Human Services] wanted us to do in planning. Now it makes sense." While Perrotta believes that the federal grants can lead to "a distortion of priorities," overall "this money is really helping us build an infrastructure in epidemiology that I only dreamed about when I came here years ago. The dual nature of this money is being put to good use. Planning is crucial and we're able to do it, and we are building new relationships with the emergency preparedness people in other departments."

Perrotta points out that Texas was using the money not just "to build the infrastructure in local and regional health departments" where epidemiologic response teams were established for bioterrorism but also "for other public health problems. Thirty-two people have been hired in the eight regional offices, which is key, and local health departments have hired two to three times that number of people." Perrotta believes that the state has been "dramatically improving its capacity and ability to respond" to bioterrorist threats as well as to other infectious disease threats, such as the West Nile virus and SARS. "It is a nice time to be in my position."

Although there was a "great interest in the legislature in the activities of government to protect public health," Perrotta's "priorities have been overwhelmed by bioterrorism, with 90 percent of my time spent on the two bioterrorism grants and smallpox." Perrotta worries that "the state department would be required to do disease surveillance and other public health activities" in the many counties that had no local health department. The basic infrastructure needed to be reinforced before more complex systems were put in place. For example, having a system of syndromic surveillance would be useful, "but," he admits, "with the resources I have, I need to worry about much more basic stuff."

Perrotta's experience as the state epidemiologist is very different from that of Jack Colley, the state coordinator of the Division of Emergency Management. In a word, Colley believes that his "budget is not adequate" to match the effort the state put into planning and preparedness operations: "You will never be able to determine the cost of the effort that we have put into it. We cannot put a dollar amount on the pure effort. September 11 changed our whole operation." Right after 9/11, "we were told that Congress was going to appropriate $3.5 billion for emergency preparedness that would go to the locals and the states. They promised $335 million in a supplemental budget to plan for how to use the $3.5 billion." Colley recalls that state employees "worked hard in the spring and developed many, many programs. We spent endless hours doing our homework. It was a tremendous effort to come together for a common cause, and there was no infighting, we were all in this together. . . . But the $3.5 billion has yet to appear, and the $335 million was reduced to $100 million. The check is in the mail but has not been delivered." In an article in *Washington Technology*, William Welsh noted that President Bush's "2003 budget promised $3.5 billion for new first-responder grants to be overseen by the Federal Emergency Management Agency. But in the bill approved by Congress, only a fraction of the money is actually new funding, according to an analysis by the National Governors Association of Washington. Most of the funds come from older programs that either have been eliminated or consolidated, or whose scope has been broadened to include homeland security, the association said."[70]

Colley explains why the failure of the federal government to deliver on its promises was so devastating: "When we prepare for terrorism, we prepare for everything." Unlike public health officials, who concentrated on infectious disease outbreaks, Colley was involved in planning for a wide range of threats to population health. Between the summer of 2002 and April 2003, he notes, Texas went "through four presidentially declared disasters," including one flood that affected forty-one counties — an area larger than that of South Carolina. In addition, much time, expense, and effort was spent gathering materials and evidence across a wide swath of the state after the Columbia shuttle disaster in February 2003. The emergency response team is "in constant response mode. . . . I'm disappointed that the federal government has not given more resources to state and local governments. Partnership should be about not just sharing information but sharing resources. The intention is there, but show me the money." Colley asserts that the establishment of the Department of Homeland Security in June 2002 further drained "resources that would have or could have gone to the states." Unlike Dennis Perrotta, who believes that bioterrorism money strengthened public health in Texas, Colley questions whether emergency preparedness money was improving emergency preparedness in Texas, and he fears that the emergency response to hurricanes, floods, and other natural disasters has been shortchanged. He worries, "FEMA [the Federal Emergency Management Agency] was a very efficient organization, but they have been brought into the Department of Homeland Security. We need to make sure that these programs stay viable in 2004."

Just as it was in public health, the relative poverty of rural county governments was a matter of concern in emergency preparedness. The Texas Association of Counties points out,

> For many counties low on funding, [preparing for terrorist attacks] could be a large order to fill. The state's Division of Emergency Management reported local governments need $195 million to better equip first responders such as police, public health, fire departments and hazardous materials teams with protective suits, decontamination equipment, and monitoring and detecting equipment. The DEM also reported there is a training shortfall among emergency responders with more than 290,000 personnel across the state in need of terrorism response training. It's safe to say that this shortfall lies largely within rural counties. Large, urban counties likely have a terrorism task force or a hazmat response team, while in a rural county the closest hazmat team might be 100 miles away and the county depends on neighboring counties for assistance and equipment.[71]

Although metropolitan areas that participated in bioterrorist preparedness activities had received federal subsidies for several years, Texas and other states considered the help inadequate. Their varied experiences with the federal grant programs, which we explore in chapter 3, are explained in part by the differences among regions and states.

Distortions Caused by Federal Bioterrorism Funding

While many state officials saw the federal involvement in bioterrorism and emergency preparedness as generally beneficial or at least a mixed blessing, American Public Health Association Executive Director Georges Benjamin (then president of the Association of State and Territorial Health Officials) and others became highly critical of how federal funding for bioterrorism was affecting population health. Within months of the World Trade Center disaster, George W. Bush proposed a budget that cut the federal allocation to prevent chronic disease, promote health, and control infectious disease (by $67 million); spending would be flat in many other programs — including, according to the *New York Times*, "childhood immunization, environmental health, preventing birth defects, and sexually transmitted diseases, including AIDS." Public health officials "not[ed] that just five Americans have been killed by bioterrorism over the last year, while thousands die each year of chronic illnesses and infectious diseases." Benjamin warned, "We will be very concerned if we are funding one thing at the expense of another," and added: "If you really want to push people towards better health, you have got to keep these programs in place." In the eyes of Marsha Martin, executive director of AIDS Action, the proposal clearly signaled that "our nation's public health has fallen off the administration's radar screen." Martin argued for broadening the definition of homeland security to include "investing in prevention and care services for people at risk and living with H.I.V."[72]

Benjamin was also concerned that federal officials, in their panicked and erratic reactions, were sending out mixed messages about future funding and priorities; he pointed out that throughout its history, public health has been plagued by "yo-yo funding." Oklahoma's former health commissioner, Leslie M. Beitsch, was equally wary: "I think it's a very significant commitment, but the question then becomes, is it a long-term commitment?"[73] Other state health officials echoed these fears. In Connecticut, hospital and health care professionals expressed concerns that despite the promises of adequate supplies, the National Pharmaceutical Stockpile (renamed in 2003 the Strategic National Stockpile) would not be there when it was needed. Norma Gyle, deputy commissioner of the Department of Public Health, feels little certainty that the "forty-two local clinics that are being organized and have been extremely active in recruiting and staffing" will have funding in future years. In Minnesota, Lee Greenfield, former legislative leader and now senior health adviser to the Hennepin County (Minneapolis) Board of Supervisors, believes that the conflicting messages about the funding for emergency preparedness would lead the "sheriff's people" to demand "space suits" for bioterrorism activities, while public health departments would go without: "Priorities were kind of mixed up."[74] Iowa officials concluded that existing programs were already suffering because of the new priorities. As of April 2003, explains Mary Kramer, president of the Iowa State Senate, they had to "tak[e] money out of other programs" because they had not received crucial funding: "We are shifting maternal and child health to the Medicaid side of the equation. We are borrowing people from the University of Iowa because it has a lot of talent that we can draw on to create a response team and do training." She complains, "We have top-down communication but no process by which to activate it."

When Angela Coron, associate director of the California Department of Health Services, was asked if her state was paying enough attention to the everyday issues of public health, she answered, "No. We are dealing with bioterrorism where the threat is unknown versus other issues where we know they are killing people. We always question where we put our limited resources." She acknowledges that "without the new bioterrorism grants from the federal government, we would not have been able to do what we have done. To do more, we need more money. We do not have enough funds to do all the things we know we need to do."

EFFECTS OF BUDGET CRISES ON PUBLIC HEALTH AND EMERGENCY PREPAREDNESS

Whatever the disagreements among state officials about the overall impact of federal bioterrorism money, there was a broad consensus that the budget problems that most states began to suffer in 2002 weakened states' abilities to respond to both bioterrorism and population health needs. The positive effects of the increased federal funding were undermined by the economic downturn that threw most state budgets into disarray, and the distortions in services and attention created by an infusion specifically aimed at bioterrorism were amplified as state legislatures attempted to cope with huge deficits and falling tax revenues. We noted in chapter 1 that the beginnings of an economic recession in 2001 were exacerbated by the stock market decline and the effects of terrorist attacks on September 11. As John M. Colmers, Scott D. Pattison, and Sheila Peterson explain, "the recession itself also stimulated countercyclical spending by states as citizens unemployed as a result of the recession or the jobless recovery that followed it turned to their state governments for assistances." As a result, "leaders of the executive and legislative branches in the states" had to "make difficult decisions in order to balance their budgets, as 49 states are constitutionally required to do."[75]

In all but a handful of states, officials complain that federal mandates requiring an increase in spending for targeted programs — mandates that were sometimes, as in the case of the campaign for smallpox vaccination, arguably ill-conceived — are at least partly responsible for cutbacks in essential public health services. A few have gone so far as to question the benefit of redirecting attention and resources, asking whether "greater resources build sustained, integrated systems that will solve problems."[76] In this section we will describe the experiences of the various states and the effect of growing deficits on public and population health programs. As months passed and shock over the events of fall 2001 faded, population health preparedness became one of a number of competing budget priorities that legislators had to consider in tough fiscal times.

In midwestern states such as Minnesota and Iowa, downturns in the economy were made worse by September 11 and the broad recession that continued into 2003. "In Iowa we have done much difficult cutting in the past three years because our revenues have been down," Mary Kramer observes. "Our economy is just stagnant." In Minnesota, Lee Greenfield notes, "the immediate effect of 9/11 was most seen in the airport and air travel" industries. The state is the home of Northwest Airlines, and mass "layoffs occurred here, as generally in the country. A lot of people are choosing not to fly. That had a serious economic effect on everything at once." In 2003, Minnesota had a $27 billion biennial budget and faced a $4.2 billion shortfall without any hope of increasing revenues, since the newly elected governor had run "on a platform of no new taxes." Further, the state "house Republicans were also elected on that basis, and they are the majority in the house. . . . Obviously, without any new taxes the proposal from the governor's office is to essentially cut $4.2 billion in spending." Since the governor had vowed not to cut public education from kindergarten through twelfth grade, Greenfield points out, "that throws it all to the rest" — including population health programs, which consumed a sizable portion of state spending. In fact, virtually all state agencies, including education, suffered serious cuts.[77] The combination of budget cuts, new federal money, and departments' changing goals left most states with fewer workers than they needed. What Mary Selecky, Washington State's secretary of health, observed in her state was repeated across the country: "the same people doing many things — no matter the funding."[78]

Arizona's state budget deficit in 2003 was $500 million, or 8 percent of the budget, and in 2004 the deficit was more than 10 percent.[79] In California Angela Coron notes the chasm between revenues and expenditures: "Our budget deficit is $34 billion, which is larger than the actual budgets of any state except New York." By June 2003, the projected shortfall was $38.2 billion,[80] adding to citizens' anger at the governor and helping to fuel a recall effort that succeeded in October. At the other end of the country, New England states were also in dire straits. In Maine, a fairly large state geographically with a small but highly dispersed rural population, $1 billion was cut from the $6 billion two-year budget in 2003. "We've been losing federal money," notes Charlene Rydell, the health policy adviser to U.S. Representative Tom Allen and formerly an influential state representative.[81] The situation in Massachusetts was equally grim. According to State Senator Harriette Chandler, a member of the health care committee, the state was "between a rock and a hard place. . . . If we're talking last year and this year — last [fiscal] year being the [calendar] year we are currently in [i.e., 2003] — I'd bet the budget has been cut 20 to 25 percent easily. On top of that there will be more cuts coming. We're $3 billion in deficit for 2004."

Only Wyoming and North Dakota reported that their state economies and budgets were in good shape. Florida and Arkansas had no budget deficits in fiscal year 2003 but had substantial deficits in FY 2004. Sheila Peterson of the North Dakota Office of Management and Budget described the state's budget as "tight but balanced. North Dakota's economy does not tend to experience the wide fluctuations, the major ups and downs, like other states' economies. In fact, as an energy-exporting and commodity-exporting state, we tend to run countercyclical to the national economy."

Overall, the economic problems of the states were immense. The Trust for America's Health, a nonprofit, nonpartisan organization, studied public health spending by states for fiscal years 2003 and 2004. More than half the states saw their budgets for public health decline in FY 2003; fifteen states suffered further declines in FY 2004, and fifteen others had their public health budgets increase by 3 percent or less.[82] In a detailed analysis of state health expenditures before and after 9/11, carried out on behalf of the National Association of State Budget Officers and the Reforming States Group, John M. Colmers, Scott D. Pattison, and Sheila Peterson found that "under the most difficult budgetary pressures in a generation, escalating health care costs for the poor and frail trumped the repair of a decaying public health infrastructure in statehouses around the country." Although "total state health expenditures grew from $271 billion in FY 2000 to $358 billion in 2003," most of this $86 billion increase "is attributable to Medicaid spending ($66 billion), which by itself is the largest share of state health spending"; population health spending represents only 5.4 percent of the total. They conclude that the states' fiscal distress and their increased Medicaid expenses "trumped the states' ability to improve the infrastructure of population health. The important but unglamorous categories of infectious disease prevention, chronic disease control and population health infrastructure will have to wait for budget increases until the economy recovers sufficiently to generate substantial increases in tax receipts."[83] Although the budget crises of the past couple of years have eased, the long-term trend is for money to remain tight, largely because of the need to fund the Medicaid and Medicare programs.[84]

The effects of these budget cuts on public health departments and programs were severe, especially in those states that had invested a significant amount of their own money in building up population health programs. Ironically, states that had relied entirely on federal grant funding suffered less when deficits forced a contraction of state health services.

In Minnesota some of the health department's signature programs were threatened. The suits against the five major tobacco companies, first initiated in 1994 by the attorneys general of Mississippi, West Virginia, and Minnesota, had resulted in the creation of what was to be a permanent endowment "to pay for antismoking campaigns for young people and for some medical education and the like." About $1.3 billion, Lee Greenfield estimates, was to be put aside. But because of the budget deficits and the state's unwillingness to raise taxes, "the governor is undoing those endowments or at least suggesting they be undone" to provide a quarter of the money needed to close the budget deficit. The rest was being accomplished through cuts, "including some severe cuts in the various programs we have for providing health care for people."

Minnesota, Greenfield points out, with its long tradition of populist politics, had developed in the mid-1970s the nation's "only statewide general assistance medical care program for adults without children who would otherwise not be eligible for Medicaid." Then in 1992, "Minnesota Care was enacted to subsidize health insurance for working families (with and without children) whose incomes were above Medicaid eligibility and who paid premiums on a sliding fee scale. . . . The part that's for families and singles without children is being drastically cut, in fact eliminated." He estimates that "about 68,000 people . . . would lose their current coverage in state or federal programs." Traditional public health activities are also being affected, despite the influx of federal money for emergency preparedness and bioterrorism. "There is nothing being eliminated," Greenfield acknowledges, but inspections of restaurants, nursing homes, and other establishments are being reduced.

In Connecticut the state has ordered 5 to 10 percent across-the-board budget cuts, notes Norma Gyle. "Lots of lab people are taking early retirement — not because of 9/11 but because of the budget crisis. We have had to cut back and there is only one manager left at the lab, and eight have retired." In Ohio the Public Health Department budget was cut 21 to 25 percent, and the effects were felt in every area. Like Minnesota, Ohio could not touch education, which here was protected by a court order rather than by campaign promises. As a result, Anne Harnish recounts, "We've had staff reductions of sixty of three hundred people approximately. Maternal child health clinics have been reduced, hemophilia treatments for adults have been eliminated, immunizations and laboratories have been cut, and local environmental health efforts have been reduced." The department has seen increases in funding in only two areas: vector-borne diseases (spurred by worries about West Nile outbreaks) and vital statistics (supported by increased fees for those specific services).

Virginia's "very large deficit" has resulted in the "yo-yo funding" that Georges Benjamin feared. According to Lisa Kaplowitz, the state's deputy commissioner for emergency preparedness and response, in 2002 "more money was put in to fund epidemiological positions and emergency medical services, but [in 2003] much money was cut because of a $2 billion deficit." Public health was able to "support its core missions," and "care for women and children, HIV, immunization, etc. have been preserved." What suffered were nonprofit agencies, which in more prosperous periods would have received state funds.

In Kentucky the budget had an 8 percent shortfall; and when the General Assembly was unable to pass a budget, the governor put together "a spending plan" that cut all departments by 10 percent. As a result, according to Rice Leach, the department of health was left "with no wiggle room at all. We used to have money to implement good new ideas, but no more." Even worse, the department "lost forty positions out of four hundred, and there is a hiring freeze." In his view, public health agencies should be anticipating future problems by undertaking septic tank and restaurant inspections, tracking outbreaks of food-borne illness, and the like, "but now we are working only on urgent problems, not routine monitoring, and things will happen if we don't keep an eye on routine monitoring." And those "things" have him deeply worried; in his years in public health (since 1966), Leach says, "This is the first time I can't maneuver to head off perceived problems like a meningitis outbreak or other acute issues." Kentucky can no longer provide the same level of service. He explains, "Maternal and child health doctors were reassigned to bioterrorism so that there was not a net loss of personnel to the department, but there was one person gone from maternal and child health."

Kansas faced a particularly difficult period. Melvin Neufeld says that "charity clinics are being overrun," following the severe economic downturn and the loss of tens of thousands of jobs in the aircraft industry that provided good health benefits. He adds, "There are also substantial cuts in Medicaid reimbursement and a lot of resistance from the provider community and threats to reduce provision of services." Cuts in residency programs for physicians may affect services to 137,000 individual patients. If its indirect costs are no longer covered by Medicare, "medical education in Kansas is threatened with collapse." Neufeld believes that the ultimate outcome will be fewer physicians in private practice and in local hospitals; as a result, "charity clinics will be even more overrun." As in other states, "the governor vowed not to cut education, so the rest of government appropriations are collapsing." Neufeld notes that the State Children's Health Insurance Program "may not have enough money to meet their matching costs, and therefore the state might have to give up all [its] federal money." As a state representative, he worries about the wide-ranging effects of subtle demographic and economic changes on the funding of medical services and institutions.

In Maine, Charlene Rydell is similarly sensitive to the broader impact on population health of the "hundreds of millions of dollars" that need to be pared from the state budget: "They are cutting funding to providers; they're cutting the number of state workers; they're cutting the university; they're changing the way state purchases are done. They're cutting incentive payments to doctors for children's health visits." Rydell explains that the state had expected more help from the federal government to do "more preparation" for emergency preparedness, "especially in hard fiscal times." Maine is "suffering from both hard economic times and heightened needs for homeland security," which impose added expenses that local communities and the state lack the resources to cover. For example, airports are now a federal responsibility, but "local police have to be at the airports more, and they are a local responsibility." The ripple effects of what initially appear to be small additions in responsibility are far-reaching: "So we're taking police off the streets to be at the airports. This will cost more money either in overtime or in more police. And where are we going to get the money? The federal presence at the airport is very visible, but people are less aware of the uniformed and plainclothes police who are also there." Rydell points out that more money for first responders was supposed to have been supplied by the Department of Homeland Security, and the lack of the expected grants has further strained "already stretched budgets. We have had to spend more money to make sewers, water, etc. more secure."

Massachusetts State Senator Harriette Chandler is also mindful of the substantial impact of budget deficits on social programs, hospital care, and other population health programs throughout her state. All are likely to be slashed, given the antitax platform espoused by the governor and much of the state legislature. "The Department of Health, according to our governor's budget, is going to be totally reorganized with major cuts," Chandler and Tim Daly, her executive assistant, report. The governor has the constitutional power "to cut unilaterally in certain areas, and health and human services is one of those areas that he can cut. That is exactly what has happened here. So we have seen over and over again hits to public health." Among the services that have been seriously affected are nursing and school-based clinics, which "in many cases are gone." In addition, research has been severely restricted, and "some of our AIDS programs have been tremendously cut — 35, maybe even 40 percent. The cuts are enormous."

Daly laments the devastating consequences for health-related programs, many of them with proven records of success: "Tobacco control has basically been eliminated. We had a model program nationally and that's gone. Absolutely gone. Hepatitis research, cancer research, any funding that was disease-specific, is gone. We have a new commissioner of public health, and I would assume that she will see her budget dramatically, dramatically cut." In short, according to Chandler, "It is a nightmare." After her nine years in the legislature, for "the first time people come up to me and say, 'I'm so glad I'm not you. There are terrible, terrible things you have to deal with this year.' And they are terrible. We've cut Medicaid so that we have turned loose on the street without health care 50,000 Medicaid patients. We suspect more will be coming. I don't know what's going to happen to these folks without preventive health care. They are going to jam our hospital ERs, and those hospitals are already teetering on financial disaster."

Chandler worries that the original commitment to public health and emergency management expressed so strongly in the immediate aftermath of the September 11 tragedy is waning: "As the days and the weeks passed since 9/11, I think the terror and the horrific impact that we had on that day and for such a long time after is receding in our minds, and so we go about our lives, and of course we've been overtaken now with this incredible budget crisis that we have. That has become, unfortunately, our first priority. So everything becomes secondary to that." Even public safety programs that appear critical to the national agenda are being cut. She points to an example: "We have an emergency medical system that we passed into the law in 2000 called EMS 2000 . . . and everybody hails it as a wonderful thing." But it, too, has been stripped of funds — "In the governor's budget this year, he cut every penny from that line. . . . We have no way of rerouting ambulances to another hospital if a hospital is closed or [an] ER is filled. We have people in the rural areas who don't have hospitals nearby — I don't know what they are going to do without a communication system. In the case of a terrorist attack, I don't know what will happen if we depend on ambulances that have no interactive communication. And that is exactly where we are because of the budget."

The enormous budget shortfall in California has already been mentioned, and the effects on public health were widespread. According to Angela Coron, in early 2003 Governor Gray Davis proposed slicing $4.5 billion from the health department's general immunization program, "and Republicans are looking at between $700 million and $1 billion more." Even in Texas, where it seemed to Dennis Perrotta to be "a nice time to be in my position," critical services have suffered, including chronic-disease surveillance, detection of birth defects, cancer care, and other areas. He sees in the legislature's planned 12 percent budget cut "a profound threat to the invisible but real public health planning, assessment, and protection services." While bioterrorism is "federally funded and not being cut," the "hepatitis and cancer registry are on the chopping block."

Local health departments were also facing budget cuts, often passed through to them from the states. In Nashville, Tennessee, for example, Robert Eadie, deputy director of the city's Metropolitan Health Department, notes that while the department has not yet felt the brunt of what he called the state's "huge budget crisis," his colleagues were worried about the possibilities of grants that might not be renewed, staff cuts in the future, and further cutbacks.[85] Similarly, Arizona projects a 10 percent difference between actual revenues and projected income, which has led public health officials to fear for their various programs. Since "there is never any discretion in taking federal money and [using these funds] for other services" that are in danger of being cut, there is a great deal of anxiety about the upcoming budget. Catherine Eden thinks "we'll be okay — but every time you pick up a paper, there is a story regarding layoffs."

J. Thomas Schedler, a state senator in Louisiana, points to the distinctive problems of a very poor state trying to balance its books, even before Katrina. He estimates that the state will face "only about a $300 to $400 million budget deficit." But because "a huge portion of our budget is dedicated," the only major areas that are not off-limits are health and hospitals, social services, and higher education. The governor has "pretty much by executive order disallowed any cuts to higher education," which means that "social services and health and hospitals take the brunt every time we get into a financial crisis." Since social service and health care are often funded through a three-to-one federal match, a $400 million reduction by the state results in a total loss of $1.6 billion, magnifying the cut's impact. The health system, broadly conceived, has thus been put under enormous stress. Schedler observes that hospitals, Medicaid reimbursement, mental institutions, and the availability of and access to pharmaceuticals and services are all threatened in a state with a large poor and uninsured population. In December 2001 the Bush administration proposed revising the hospital reimbursement system with the expectation of saving the federal government $9 billion over the course of five years — a change that would result in putting a larger burden on state budgets.[86] Schedler points out that Louisiana has "a fairly high Medicaid population. . . . With the economy being what it is and the cost of health care, we are seeing a tremendous number of people who are now 'the working uninsured,'" a number pushed up by the combination of layoffs, reductions in health benefits by employers, and decisions by the "younger population who are taking risks in going without insurance." He notes that "almost across the board our institutions — developmental centers, mental institutions, and hospitals — have taken a 15 percent cut," including 15 percent cuts in pharmaceuticals, for example, at the very time that there has been "an 18 to 19 percent rapid growth in our pharmacy bills with Medicaid."

Louisiana's extensive charity hospital system, begun under Huey Long in the 1930s, is facing its own crisis. At the same time that demand for services from the charity system is increasing, according to Schedler, people are asking, "Should we disband that system? . . . There is a raging debate in Louisiana [over whether] . . . we are the smartest people on earth now or the stupidest. We haven't determined which one yet." The state, unlike local governments, cannot collect property taxes, and it thus has few options for increasing revenues to fund the hospital system. And because six of the ten charity hospitals around the state are teaching hospitals, "when you start monkeying with this . . . you also monkey with the education of our health professionals." Private hospitals, of course, would resist taking on more patients without full reimbursement. Since many of the charity hospitals are "economic engines" for local communities, any reduction in their support raises the number of unemployed and therefore the number of uninsured in the state. "It's really a monumental problem," Schedler declares.

THE SMALLPOX CAMPAIGN AND POPULATION HEALTH PROGRAMS

Even as state budget crises were threatening public health departments around the country with disruption at best and disaster at worst, the smallpox vaccination campaign, initiated in December 2002, put added strains on the system. On the one hand, the federal program to inoculate half a million health care workers, the first step in what was projected to be a three-stage process, drew national attention to public health and its needs. Citizens were reminded of the enormous effort required to ensure that their water, air, and food are safe. In this context, as the United States began to mobilize for war against Iraq and as the likelihood of the Iraqis' using biological agents was discussed, support for a national campaign to prepare for a possible smallpox attack was widespread. But as the smallpox vaccination campaign continued and it became clear that it was actually draining resources and energies from population health initiatives in the states rather than strengthening them, that support quickly began to evaporate. Some officials praised the effort as a stimulus to readying the country for possible future bioterrorist events, but soon lack of commitment in the public health community, resistance among the general public, and the refusal of many health providers to volunteer for vaccination in effect stopped the campaign in its tracks.

From the first, states mobilized to organize broad inoculation campaigns directed at state and local health care workers. The initial step, recalls Angela Coron, was to develop methods for conferring with officials in "all health jurisdictions at one time"; those officials "utilized e-mail and conference calls to dialogue with each other about concerns about the CDC guidelines and their implementation at the local level." In California they proceeded cautiously, phasing in their system in February 2003. "We waited until, as a state, we were ready and provided training for localities"; once there was confidence that personnel were well organized, "we began shipping vaccine." In Arizona the state was methodical in organizing its campaign, even though neither the governor nor the director of the Department of Health Services supported the smallpox program or encouraged hospital staff or others to be vaccinated.[87] Catherine Eden and David Engelthaler describe the approach to inoculation as "very cautious. . . . There has been a lot of planning, a lot of people participating in getting a system put together in Arizona."

Norma Gyle remembers that in Connecticut the response of local health authorities to the campaign was "excellent." Eden recalls that in Arizona, many believed that even though "the possibility of an intentional release of smallpox virus is remote, . . . the consequences of a release would be so serious that the state must be ready." Similarly, Lisa Kaplowitz in Virginia notes an initial "good response from the health department."[88] In Louisiana and New Jersey, health officers agreed, there was at first little opposition and a fair amount of enthusiasm for the effort to inoculate health care workers throughout the states.[89]

But despite the early optimism and careful planning, many, if not most, of the states began to encounter resistance to the campaign for a variety of reasons. As of June 2003, the goal of vaccinating half a million people was far from being met. Only 37,608 health care workers had received the vaccine, according to reports presented at a conference called by the CDC.[90] In California, for example, the goal of the campaign's first stage was 40,000, but according to Angela Coron the state had inoculated only "somewhat over 1,000" by the end of March. One of the major issues in California and other states was the safety of the vaccine itself. Systematic vaccination against smallpox had ended in the United States in 1972, and the small but actual risk of the vaccine seemed to many to outweigh the benefit of being protected from a hypothetical attack.

Minnesota quickly "ran into some trouble with some of our doctors," says Lee Greenfield, as evidence surfaced that the vaccine could create problems for people with heart disease. In Ohio, too, according to Anne Harnish, there were concerns about potential heart problems, as well as worries "about spreading the live virus to AIDS patients," who might be particularly vulnerable because their immune systems were compromised. Some infectious-disease doctors in the state feared possible outbreaks of smallpox as vaccinated patients shed the live virus, even though the vaccine contains not smallpox itself but vaccinia (a related virus) and thus cannot infect any individual with the disease. In Texas Dennis Perrotta, the "architect" of the program there, had "grave concerns about inoculating large numbers of people." When asked by a local paper whether he would be vaccinated, he answered, "I will be immunized, and I will live someplace else for three weeks (while the vaccination site sheds virus)," because his wife's eczema made her particularly susceptible to complications from exposure to vaccinia.[91] Perrotta remembers that "people throughout Texas asked, 'What is the risk? What is the chance of smallpox?'" and the "hospital staff asked, 'Should I be inoculated if I don't know the risk [of other health consequences]?'" The state had estimated that phase 1 would require 40,000 doses of vaccine, but by mid-April only 2,700 had been vaccinated. In Kentucky, as well as in Virginia and Arizona, fear of the vaccine's side effects weakened the campaign.[92]

Worries about the safety of the vaccine merged with other anxieties circulating through the country. In some communities, both a general distrust of government among various segments of the population and a particular distrust of immunizations created wariness about the campaign. Lee Greenfield in Minnesota noted at the time "another strange movement" that was interfering with the campaign: "There are a whole bunch of folks who go to the legislature protesting against immunizations, period. Why should kids have them?" He believes that many are searching for reasons to reject inoculation, and "they read the data backward. It's really strange," he remarks. "They talk about the one person in a million who has problems with the vaccine and not the hundreds of thousands who would get sick. . . . There is a movement against vaccinations. People argued, 'We don't need this. Are you going to force us to be immunized?'" He finds them hard to label, calling them "this funny group of people who are anti-immunization or . . . anti–[organized] medicine . . . they believe in alternatives. They're sort of mixed together in funny ways. I don't think it's very well organized. But they have had an impact with the legislature." Greenfield points out that these antivaccinationists do not fit into traditional political categories: "It's the far left and the far right together. I mean it's the most absurd companions you could imagine." Some believe that "we're putting something in the vaccines to control them," while others see the vaccination program as a conspiracy of the drug companies.

Similarly, in Missouri Ronald Cates notes that the campaign elicited a strange alliance of individuals from the "extreme left and extreme right [who] are so extreme they touch each other." The antivaccinationists "thought that the government was putting something in the vaccine to control them. Some were scared that people in black helicopters were swooping down and worried that surveillance equaled helicopters." Perrotta says that some in Texas feared that this was a forced vaccination program but "were mollified when they found out it was voluntary." Others in the Lone Star State were "concerned about the overarching power of the federal government," but he told them not to worry since "these are the people that brought us Amtrak."

Many public health personnel, embroiled in horrific budget fights, were troubled by a more practical issue: the cost of the campaign. In Minnesota, says Greenfield, the health department organized a campaign to immunize "key people, . . . [but] the costs of that were astronomical per person [because] it was a small number of people." Maine, too, found "the costs of the vaccination campaign" worrisome, according to Charlene Rydell. "We need to pay [temporary hospital workers] to take over from people who are vaccinated and need to be isolated from sick patients. But we don't have extra people and a reservoir of people who can take over." If state officials had been convinced there was an imminent danger, the response might have been different. But in Maine, she says, such was not the case. "There is not a strong enough threat at this time, especially when we're having budget problems, and we're getting resistance from individuals especially with publicity about health problems and deaths. The federal government has not come through with funds for the true costs of the program, . . . about $200 per person when there are no complications." In Maine, Rydell points out, individuals in every level of the health system appeared to be resisting the smallpox inoculation campaign. "Hospitals are private, and there are no health care professionals being vaccinated. We're not getting many volunteers from the health care community. We have put together a plan, if in fact the threat is more real than it appears to be now. People are worried about the costs, and nobody is paying us to do it."

Financial concerns also underlay the unwillingness of health care professionals and hospitals to participate in the program. Many institutions were apprehensive about being held liable if someone who was inoculated fell sick or died, or if patients became ill as a result of being exposed to hospital staff who had been in contact with recently vaccinated individuals. Staff members themselves worried that they might not be covered by workers' compensation if they became ill after receiving an inoculation. Gene Matthews, then legal advisor to the CDC and now director of the Institute of Public Health Law at Georgia State University, believes that "there were three concerns: liability, compensation, and risk assessment (do we really need to be doing this?); these issues got mixed up with each other as we tried to implement it."[93] "State and local authorities made clear," says Joseph Henderson, who is now CDC senior management official to the New York State Department of Health and was formerly the CDC's chief of program operations for bioterrorism preparedness and response, that "from the beginning there would be problems because we did not have the compensation issue resolved and we did not have the liability issue resolved." These questions took months to resolve and generated much tension, and some states — including Washington — refused to vaccinate anyone until they were. Indeed, Nevada still will not vaccinate at all.[94]

Ed Thompson, then the chief of public health improvement in the CDC's Office of the Director and now chief of the CDC's Public Health Practice, argues that "there was uneven acceptance of the smallpox program. Some states embraced it even if they did it reluctantly. Most states understood that it needed to be done. Immediately following 9/11 ASTHO called on the Department of HHS to radically expand production of the vaccine. But HHS was already in the process of doing it. Smallpox was one of the scariest issues because we could not protect the population." Thompson points to another factor that may have interfered with the program's implementation: the linking of the smallpox campaign with the buildup to the invasion of Iraq, he believes, undercut support for the effort in some areas of the country while aiding the effort in others. "In some areas [e.g., the Southeast], patriotism generated very hard work. Almost as a part of the war effort. In other areas, their participation was hampered because they felt the Iraq war and smallpox were interrelated. In the Northeast, because liberals were suspicious of the war effort, it hampered their support for the smallpox campaign."[95]

In Minnesota and other states, a number of hospitals "opted out" because of their worries about how involvement would affect their bottom line.[96] Many hospitals were concerned that being designated the emergency smallpox hospital for an area could bring financial ruin if patients, fearing exposure, chose to go elsewhere. Lisa Kaplowitz told a reporter that more than half of Virginia's hospitals that provide emergency services refused to participate until their concerns about compensation and liability had been met.[97] Even in Kentucky, where Rice Leach, as the public health commissioner, "was the first in the state to receive the vaccine," "the compensation issue is a real problem, a much bigger problem than fear of bad reactions to inoculations."[98] In mid-November 2002 a survey "found that 16 of 84 hospitals said they weren't certain whether they would prevaccinate employees. Most wanted more information, [Leach] said."[99]

Dennis Perrotta found real resistance in certain Texas hospitals. He recalls some administrators saying, "We want to participate, but we want a letter absolving us of all responsibility" — something the state could not do. He worried about the other side of the issue: What would happen if "a hospital had someone come in with smallpox — wouldn't they be liable if other people got infected and they hadn't done anything to protect them beforehand?" In Tennessee opposition from hospitals as well as personnel was strong, especially at the Vanderbilt University

Medical Center, a level 1 trauma center. Robert Eadie, a local health official with extensive knowledge of statewide events, found this refusal to take part in the program especially troubling because the emergency room personnel would be first to see this type of problem.

State Senator Harriette Chandler is also well aware of the resistance of professional staff to the inoculation campaign in Massachusetts. She recalls, "The nurses and doctors have been very unwilling to cooperate, particularly the nurses. . . . That is not something that is original to us. I think this is happening elsewhere as well, all across the country." The nurses "are afraid that they are going to get sick. I think that's what it really comes down to." Furthermore, the state has no capability to cover the "liability for anyone who contracts smallpox in the course of inoculation." As a result, Chandler believes, "we are going to continue to see those nurses unwilling to participate, and without them we can't." In Arizona, according to Catherine Eden, some "hospitals came out front saying they would not participate in the prevaccination program." She continues, "We were not trying to get every hospital to participate. Our goal was to have public health teams and select health care teams . . . be vaccinated around the state. But there has been resistance," particularly from public health workers and hospitals, arising from the workers' compensation issue. "We don't have a large number of people vaccinated because of those concerns and because we have concerns about causing ill effects on the public's health."

Georges Benjamin notes that in March 2003, the administration put out a compensation bill that was very "different from what the public health community desires. We want no caps and no delay before being reimbursed for health care issues. But this is going to be a political process, and there is going to be give-and-take." The bill would have set a lifetime cap on compensation at $262,100, with an annual cap of the smaller of 66.6 percent of lost wages (75 percent for those with dependents) or $50,000. It failed to pass the House in late March, but a revamped version passed in mid-April and the president signed the bill into law on April 30, 2003.

"Why Are We Doing This?": The Growing Uneasiness over the Smallpox Vaccination Campaign

The uneasiness that arose among those considering the safety of the vaccine and worrying about its financial costs was a concrete manifestation, some informants assert, of a growing discomfort with the entire rationale for the smallpox campaign. Lee Greenfield of Minnesota summarized the situation: "There are a lot of people now reluctant . . . to get immunized. There is the whole public health question that people have raised. We do not know of an actual case of smallpox that exists in the world." Thus, he asked, "Why are we doing this?" Many public health administrators throughout the country felt generally that a political agenda had trumped public health judgment, and many expressed their view that public health should be left to public health professionals, rather than risk the dissemination of inaccurate messages that would undermine public confidence in their authority.

Across the United States, state administrators spoke of the distortions in program and policy caused by the smallpox campaign. In Virginia, Lisa Kaplowitz points out, county "departments of health have had to give up some of their core functions, and you can do that for a short time but not for the long term, because of this rush to do smallpox inoculations. If we go and ask the fire folks to monitor smallpox, they could turn around and say, 'You got extra money and we didn't.'" A number of state administrators saw the federal government's insistence on a smallpox campaign as an intrusion if not outright arm-twisting. As Kaplowitz reports, "To say that there was pressure from the federal government was an understatement. . . . They say they are not mandating it, but the pressure is intense." In the end, it was presented as an issue of security, not public health, but many questioned the focus on smallpox even in those terms, arguing that it was taking time and resources from defending against other pressing bioterrorist threats. She adds, "Somebody high up believes there is some likelihood that smallpox is a terrorist issue. The downside is that you're not looking out for agents that are more likely. There are a lot of other organisms that are available to many people — plague, anthrax, botulism, etc. We are not focusing on the broader issues of biological, chemical, or radiological terrorism. They're being overshadowed by smallpox."

Similarly, in California the smallpox campaign was seen as a distraction from the core functions of public health as well as more comprehensive security issues. "It has shifted our focus because we wanted to make sure we were implementing smallpox vaccination safely," Angela Coron says. "It has pulled people from the immunization program and from the broader BT program to just focus on smallpox." California had been given verbal assurances by the CDC that the state "could shift some budget from bioterrorism to smallpox, but it took a long time to get the guidelines in writing so the policy could be implemented. It was frustrating because it took much more effort than expected." Overall, because the California system is highly decentralized, "the impact on the state has been varied . . . and each jurisdiction pulled people from different programs. But immunization was pulled most extensively."

Even in states where federal money was seen as a means of buttressing the public health infrastructure in general, the emphasis on smallpox was a major distraction. The money was an "interesting double-edged sword," according to Robert Eadie. He believes that public health departments do the work essential for bioterrorism defense, because he views it as "a fancy way to say 'communicable disease control.'" But the focus on what he called the "bad news" of smallpox "took away from base services," as Tennessee spent an enormous amount of time "getting geared up for smallpox." Moreover, he wonders, "Was the effort worthwhile and needed?" The state has not changed priorities, but it "can't do as much." Employees were shifted away from its TB elimination project and its syphilis emergency project because "bioterrorism moneys were used for equipment and infrastructure instead of staff." And in Iowa, where "there has just not been a public outcry to inoculate the masses of people," Senate President Mary Kramer believes that "in the great scheme of things, the fear of smallpox is overrated." What was really needed were funds to help the state "to protect our food supply, agriculture, and act on contagious diseases. Because even if they are less deadly, they are also very debilitating." With the "laser intensity of focus on smallpox," she worries that "other threats" are being overlooked.

All these difficulties were identified very early in the planning efforts in the Midwest. In October 2002 health officials from Illinois, Indiana, Michigan, Minnesota, Ohio, and Wisconsin met in Chicago to discuss how they might coordinate and organize the smallpox vaccination campaign that had just been proposed by the federal government. The meeting was aimed at identifying the various problems that needed to be addressed even before planning for the campaign could begin. Among the "essential issues" they immediately identified were hospital and personnel "indemnification from liability for all aspects of smallpox vaccination and follow-up"; the voluntary nature of the campaign; "compensation for injury due to any contact with vaccinia virus, including compensation for furloughs and lost work time"; and logistical matters revolving around laboratory space, public education and public relations, the chain of command between federal, state, and local health officers, data management, data sharing, training, and the need to understand the "tradeoffs (diversions) of time and resources: public health infrastructure building versus administration of smallpox vaccinations."[100] Despite their efforts to anticipate potential trouble, state administrators soon found themselves dealing with most of these problems.

Georges Benjamin takes a long view of the entire recent history of bioterrorist threats. The anthrax mailings helped focus the nation on the dangerous possibility of infectious diseases as a terrorist tool and showed how an infusion of federal money could combat that threat: "Lots of money was poured in for all-hazards management to build up the public health infrastructure." But the smallpox inoculation campaign is another matter. Even though "smallpox has become the new mandate," he notes, it "has been underfunded"; furthermore, single-minded attention to it has "sacrificed core public health activities," pulling money and people from other programs. The general fight against terrorism has also been undermined, as "we have also sacrificed an all-hazards management (bioterrorism) approach to concentrate on one specific disease." Benjamin captures the general uneasiness of many in the public health community as well as in the broader population:

> Many public health practitioners believe the case for smallpox inoculation has not been effectively made and is taking away resources and personnel from things we know we should be doing. It is pulling people away from screening for HIV and the counseling of AIDS patients, prenatal care clinics, other immunizations, and inspection programs for other diseases. A basic surveillance system is already lacking. And money is being used to deal with a theoretical disease. . . . Already people are being laid off in disease and inspection programs but are being hired in bioterrorism. They are being funded by shifting moneys around. Phase 1 was supposed to inoculate 500,000 people, but only about 12,000 have been inoculated so far. It is well behind schedule, it is stalled.[101]

The program does have some success stories, as communication and coordination often improved among the public health and health care entities planning and conducting smallpox vaccinations. "The approach taken in Indiana and some other states," says Joe Hunt, assistant commissioner of information services and policy for the Indiana State Department of Public Health, "was to focus on training, clinic planning, and response coordination for prompt effective response if smallpox is reintroduced."[102] In fact, the debates over the program itself had a positive impact. As J. Nick Baird, director of the Ohio Department of Health, puts it, the smallpox debates helped "the nation move quickly to address some ascendant concerns and will stand us in good stead should we need to move quickly on an outbreak in the future." Though the federal government's goal of inoculating half a million people was questionable, the public health community "essentially decided at what level we should vaccinate for smallpox. Although the numbers may be smaller than many states desired," he notes, "we will have a cadre of persons who can respond in the event of need."[103]

Wisconsin: One Administrator's View

Wisconsin, a state with a diverse mix of urban and rural populations, populist as well as conservative political traditions, and a nationally recognized state university, makes a good case study of the ways that the aftermath of 9/11 created problems and opportunities for public health administrators.

For the Wisconsin Department of Health and Family Services, the September 11 attacks and the anthrax episode just three weeks later revealed fundamental weaknesses in the state's infrastructure and limits in its ability to address public health crises. The state recognized that it had been able to cope with the growing fears within the state only by overtaxing its workforce and by filling the emergency teams with existing staff, who therefore had to abandon other public health functions. "Resource constraints" was the polite term used for what some administrators described as the "exploitation" of a dedicated workforce and the "illegal redeployment" of staff from some necessary services to the labs.[104] There were too few workers trained in epidemiology to address the many reports of possible anthrax contamination, and the few trained epidemiologists and laboratory workers were too concentrated in Madison and Milwaukee to respond adequately to reports from the more distant, rural areas of the state.[105] "We have been stretched," reported John Chapin, then administrator of the Division of Public Health and later the director of the Division of Health Care Financing in the Department of Health and Family Services; "because of capacity, DHFS can only deal with one moderate-sized event for a limited period of time." Within one week, in early October 2001, the department had had to address "both panic (anthrax) and pancakes (E. coli) at the same time. Luckily, one was false and one was small. . . . We were lucky."[106] When the anthrax scare began, headlines and local television news coverage made the public aware of the huge efforts made by this usually invisible department.

Chapin recalls the reaction of the public health community to the attention that it received in the months following the outbreak of anthrax and the federal decision to inoculate as many as 500,000 people against the threat of smallpox: "September 11 was a tragedy for the nation and the people. But it gave great hope to public health. It was the first glimpse that the federal government would truly help public health."[107] He notes that "many in the public health community . . . felt that they have been unfairly left out for a generation from the great federal and state funding frenzy of health care financing. Now, with the tragedy of recent events, many in public health view[ed] this war as the 'great opportunity' to join the frenzy." They took heart from the "wonderful policy decision" by Wisconsin's governor to exempt those in public health from a general government hiring freeze; according to Chapin, "all in DHFS declared conceptual victory: State government had finally gotten it."[108] Wisconsin had budgeted $250 million for public health, and was expecting new federal funding for bioterrorism of perhaps $20 million.[109] At that moment, it seemed that public health might be able to expand basic services, consolidate its infrastructure, and reorganize local and state bureaucracies. Mirroring a broader consensus at the national level, local administrators reveled in the visions that federal moneys might make possible: "At the local, state, and national level [there was] much talk that the 'lean' years for public health are now over. At the [2001] American Public Health Association convention, most of the hall conversation was that the national coffers would soon be open to public health because of the war and that this would solve the long-term infrastructure problems with the system."[110]

At the very least, it seemed to those in Wisconsin's planning group, the new popular, media, and federal attention to public health held out the promise that long-standing deficiencies in the health department's electronic data system, its processing of information, and its coordination of state and local health activities would be addressed; moreover, they expected assistance in developing a "sufficient and competent workforce and equitable, adequate, and stable funding." In a memo, Chapin called these "the preconditions for the health of the public health system," and administrators believed that "any funding to enhance the capacity of public health to deal with the issues of terrorism and national security need[s] to address these broad systems requirements. It [is] the capacity of the system rather than its particular focus that needs to be fixed." He pointed out that "what [was] wrong with public health [could] not be fixed in a month or a year or the duration of a war. Fixing public health [was] the work of a decade of sustained effort."[111] "True public health infrastructure development focuses on long-range, pre-incident planning in terms of increasing capacity and resilience of public health, the family, the community, and the population," he declared elsewhere.[112] "Wisconsin spent a lot of time writing a proposal," Chapin recalls, which cost the department "$1 million. . . . Fifty people contributed to writing it and consulted with scores of people in the community" as they developed 287 objectives. Ultimately, the state received $20 million for public health; the department "kept a small amount and distributed [the] rest to local and community groups and the twelve regional consortia."[113]

Genuine attention to public health would have radical implications for the state and for the country. "September 11, 2001, should have changed the . . . debate in America for the next decade," Chapin argued. "Cost containment is now secondary to the more immediate question of the health status of the population and threats to that status. Surveillance is now an issue of national security. Epidemiology, rather than economics, is the key discipline for looking at health data in a time of bioterrorism."[114] Experts agreed that increasing the capacity of and access to hospitals, boosting staff levels at local health departments, increasing Medicare and Medicaid funding, expanding mental health services, and even strengthening families and community institutions were essential for preparing the state for emergencies.[115] For administrators, there was no hard-and-fast distinction between planning for an "emergency response" and for everyday needs and services; as Chapin observes, "Actual incident response is useful only in a probability situation that is likely to be insignificant for any one locality; but pre- and post-incident infrastructure is useful every day and everywhere."[116] In briefing the Board of the Wisconsin State Lab of Hygiene at a March 2002 meeting, he emphasized that "the overriding theme for Wisconsin's plan would be 'dual-use.' General public health and disaster response, including terrorism response, suggests we should be creating a dual capacity response. The Department of Health and Family Services's approach is to build an infrastructure capable of everyday use in the public health system."[117]

Chapin's broad view of public health readiness transcends the bureaucracy itself and the traditional needs of the Wisconsin health department. In many ways he sees it as part of a broader population health program. "This funding should also include complementary health and human services, and not just public health services," he notes. Specifically, mental health services as well as "health care and human service functions outside of the Division of Health" must be addressed by planners. "One prime example is mental health assistance in terrorist events, especially as it relates to children. In the old days," Chapin argues, "mental health [w]as not . . . traditionally viewed as a 'public health' issue at the state level. . . . Family health and its relation to children's mental health are crucial to a national response to domestic terrorism. There is now another factor of violence in the lives of America's children that transcends class, race, and region." Chapin believes that "both mental health education at the community/family level as well as intervention at the family/individual level should come as a package of 'human services' that should be linked in funding to public health services. These would include mental health, housing, acute health care, employment/retraining and relocation, nutritional support, and all the other services needed to mitigate the impact of these events. These services should be managed as a single package at the community and state level. Therefore, their funding at the broadest human services federal level should be integrated."[118]

As they planned to integrate preparedness into an effort to improve ongoing services, public health administrators in Wisconsin thought the new focus on public health might be a panacea. But their early hopes were dashed by a combination of political, economic, and internal problems. The most immediate of these was the state's ongoing budget crises. The recession had driven Wisconsin's deficit above $1 billion, and what looked to the public health community like a windfall for augmenting services looked to legislators in Madison, the state capital, more like an opportunity to reduce the state's contribution to existing public health programs. In the face of competing demands from other state agencies, legislators believed that the federal funding allowed them to reduce funding because "the feds were doing it." The problem, according to Chapin, was that "money was coming to the state not for infrastructure but for short-term problems, not long-term problems," and the misplaced emphasis added greatly to the system's existing strains.[119] While the governor and some top administrators understood that a robust infrastructure was crucial to preparedness, "there [was] still only a superficial awareness of the role of public health" among many budget department legislators and administrators who wanted to focus solely on bioterrorism.[120]

Chapin points to the Bush administration's push to oust Jeffrey Koplan from the directorship of the CDC as a major turning point. He recalls that "Koplan, when he was with the CDC, talked a true message of dual capacity," recognizing the need "to build up public health infrastructure" to ensure that the states could "also be ready for bioterrorism." In insisting that public health readiness required a system of surveillance and information exchange integrated with local voluntary organizations and with ongoing public health activities, Koplan spoke for that large portion of the public health community who believed, in Chapin's words, that "if you're not using things every day, you are wasting [them]." In contrast, "the White House wanted proposals that demanded specific mandates."[121] Within a few months, according to Chapin, efforts to reform the DHFS succumbed to federal and local legislative goals.

Though state budget woes cut short the hopes for infrastructural improvements briefly raised by the anthrax scare, their effects were amplified by the campaign for smallpox inoculation, announced by President Bush on December 13, 2002, and criticized harshly by Chapin. He notes that "smallpox diverted human resources to a political event and posturing. Wisconsin had to divert money from building regional coalitions and infrastructure to get ready for inoculations." In his view, the federal government's myopic focus on bioterrorism doomed Wisconsin's effort to build a broad-based public health infrastructure that could provide both needed protection from smallpox and adequate services for the rest of the population. Although the department believed that assisting rural as well as urban areas made sense for a state with a considerable population outside its largest cities, Madison and Milwaukee, "the feds said you can't do this. We had to follow their guidelines."[122] Chapin wrote that the campaign would weaken "the long-term strength of public health at the state level" in its efforts "to defend against all sources of terrorism." Moreover, it would weaken the public "consensus about the war on terrorism because *why* we are doing it is dubious, if not bogus, outside the beltway." Since a key purpose of bioterrorism funding "is to deal with realistic and immediate credible threats from biological, chemical, radioactive, and conventional terrorism," planning for such an inoculation campaign is important. But "actually immunizing people for smallpox" when no public official could honestly argue that such an attack was imminent or even credible would undermine public confidence. Chapin worried that the campaign was cynically undertaken to bolster the administration domestically and to build support for the coming war in Iraq. He urged governors "to plan, prepare, train, and educate, but not to actually vaccinate until there is either a credible threat or a verified event in the world. There is time. The smallpox models do not predict instant world contamination as that is not how it spreads. Therefore, governors should accept the vaccines, but not implement until the what, why, how, and when makes sense."[123]

When the federal government ignored this advice, focused on smallpox, and then began the inoculation of thousands of health care workers across the country, Chapin resigned. He saw the emphasis on smallpox as a fatal diversion from building an infrastructure for population health.[124]

THE DRAFT MODEL ACT AND THE STATES

Even before the events of 9/11, a discussion about how states and their public health agencies should prepare for new and unexpected disasters was under way. The terrorist attacks had many immediate consequences — including passage of the USA PATRIOT Act, the creation of the Department of Homeland Security, the incarceration and deportation of many men of Middle Eastern descent, an expansion of federal surveillance activities, and restrictions on implementing the Freedom of Information Act — and the general mobilization against terrorism also radically transformed the jobs and focus of public health officials. Complicating their response to the new geopolitical situation and broadening the debate were what some criticized as the poor federal handling of the anthrax episode and, later, the smallpox inoculation campaign, as well as concerns about perceived threats to the rights of individuals. At the same time, decisions about bioterrorism and public health preparedness were being framed by deep worries about how the needed steps could be funded when state budgets were suffering the effects of prolonged economic stagnation.

At the behest of Gene Matthews, then legal counsel to the CDC, Lawrence Gostin and Stephen Teret at the Center for Law and the Public's Health (established in 2000 by Georgetown University and Johns Hopkins University) began in mid-2001 to draw up the Model State Emergency Health Powers Act, with input from staff of the National Conference of State Legislatures, the National Governors Association, the National Association of Attorneys General, the Association of State and Territorial Health Officials, and the National Association of County and City Health Officials. After September 11 and the anthrax outbreaks shortly thereafter, the urgency of their work greatly increased. By late October 2001, a draft model act had been posted on the Internet and started to circulate throughout the country.[125]

This act was conceived of as a template that the states could use to check their existing public health emergency laws for deficiencies. Anthony Moulton, co-director of the CDC's Public Health Law Program, notes that "the approach Gostin and his colleagues took to preparing the draft Model Act had two basic parts." The first was "to examine the existing public health laws of the states and to include provisions the authors considered exemplary." As a result the act was "largely composed of provisions of existing state laws." The second "was to include provisions the authors believed important because they comported with modern jurisprudence, for example, with the due process reforms of the Warren Court."[126]

A similar attempt had been made as recently as 1998, when the Robert Wood Johnson Foundation and the W. K. Kellogg Foundation jointly funded fourteen state-level partnerships as well as partnerships in forty-one communities and tribal jurisdictions in order to "identify, analyze, and address challenges collaboratively pertaining to public health system improvement." A major part of this project was the creation of a uniform public health law that transcended state and local jurisdictions. These efforts, called the Turning Point initiative, were administered by NACCHO and the University of Washington School of Public Health and Community Medicine.[127] But lacking the impetus of a national emergency, these attempts at coordination achieved only limited success, resulting in relatively minor adjustments in relationships and law.

Even after 9/11, a number of state legislators viewed the Model Act as tantamount to a "governmental takeover."[128] The National Conference of State Legislatures found that some of its members had "gone ballistic" when they learned that they were "being listed as a collaborator on the draft," though the group ultimately endorsed it.[129] Across the political spectrum, analysts noted, "there appeared to be no great enthusiasm for the gradual recodification foreseen when the act was first released."[130] Many comments were received during this period of public review — some supportive, some critical, many making helpful substantive and technical suggestions — and, as had always been planned, they were taken into account as the document was revised. In late December 2001, the Center for Law and the Public's Health circulated a second draft of the act.[131]

In brief, the Model Act gives governors broad authority to declare a state of emergency in the event of a bioterrorist attack. Moreover, public health officials are allowed access to personal health records without first getting the patient's consent (as is usually necessary). It requires physicians and pharmacists to report "unusual" health events and physicians to send state health departments information on individual patients who show unusual symptoms. The act also authorizes public health officials to initiate quarantine and isolation measures, to mandate vaccinations and medical examinations, and to "seize and control" personal property and access to communications. Finally, it grants governors exclusive power over "funds appropriated for emergencies" and requires that states develop comprehensive plans for responding to an attack.[132]

The Model Act focused the attention of many public health officials on serious questions about their rights — on the federal, state, and local levels — to undertake quarantine, isolation, surveillance, and other activities that might infringe civil liberties. As Lawrence Gostin argues in his important book *Public Health Law: Power, Duty, Restraint,* the Constitution contains an inherent tension between "the legal powers and duties of the state to assure the conditions for people to be healthy . . . and the limitations of the power of the state to constrain the autonomy, privacy, liberty, propriety, or other legally protected interests of individuals for the protection or promotion of community health."[133] Many who today are making or carrying out public health policy in the United States are confused about their powers and even their responsibilities as they seek to control infectious diseases. For much of the nineteenth century, as various epidemics swept through the nation's growing cities and killed large numbers of children and adults alike, few public health officials questioned their right to engage in activities that intruded on personal liberties and civil rights. But in the twentieth century, as new methods of prevention and cure dramatically reduced the prevalence and deadliness of epidemic diseases, use of forced quarantine, isolation, and involuntary removal to infectious disease hospitals almost completely stopped. With very limited exceptions — notably the advent of AIDS and the accompanying resurgence of tuberculosis during the 1980s — concerns over civil liberties had come to outweigh the perceived benefits of allowing public health officials police powers. In such a context, the Model Act became a lightning rod in the debate over how and if public health law should be revised to deal with the threats of bioterrorism and chemical attack.

In 2002 the proposed act played the role envisioned by its drafters, as most states assessed the adequacy of their own laws by comparing them to the model. "Twenty states took action on the legislation. At times it was defeated," notes Anthony Moulton. "For example, Iowa defeated a model bill in 2002 but recently adopted it." Crucial to the Model Act's success, in his view, is that "each state is shaping and tailoring it to [its] special needs," while engaging with broad concerns about civil liberties and private property rights. Questions were raised about whether the federal or a state government could come in and take over a hospital. Does the state have the right to intrude on the doctor-patient relationship? Is forced quarantine (or even isolation) a real possibility? How far should government powers extend? The legislation has created strange alliances and even stranger splits. "In most states," Moulton explains, "ACLU [American Civil Liberties Union] chapters were opposed to the Model Act; but others, such as [those in] Vermont, favored it. Some conservative administrators who helped write state legislation modeled on the act have been attacked by conservative organizations worried about increasing powers of the state."[134]

The national media reported opposition to the Model Act from groups on both the left and the right that feared the possibilities of government intrusion into the lives of ordinary Americans. Thus, in a front-page article titled "Many States Reject Bioterrorism Law; Opponents Say It's Too Invasive," *USA Today* quoted Barry Steinhardt of the ACLU, who deplored the Model Act as "giv[ing] governors and state health officials a blank check to impose the most draconian sorts of measures"; it also quoted Andrew Schlafly of the conservative Association of American Physicians and Surgeons, who charged that the act "goes far beyond bioterrorism. . . . Unelected state officials can force treatment or vaccination of citizens against the advice of their doctors."[135] Respected health ethicists also weighed in with criticism; in the prestigious *New England Journal of Medicine*, George Annas argued that there was "no empirical evidence that draconian provisions for quarantine, such as those outlined in the Model Act, are necessary or desirable."[136]

Reforming State Law

Few administrators in state or local health agencies found themselves embroiled in the broad concerns raised by civil libertarians, academics, and constitutional lawyers. Many, like Nashville's Robert Eadie, felt that it was "nice to have guidelines for recommended best practice for emergency responses"; they welcomed explicit formulations of the governor's responsibilities and the obligations and rights of public health personnel during an emergency. And if smallpox were to break out, he says, "we would need to know what to do with the infected." Could the public health authorities seize a hotel or shut down a hospital? In Tennessee, where state and local officials had been working with civil libertarians since the mid-1990s to develop communicable disease regulations, the debate about the lengths to which public health officials might go was relatively muted.

Many legislators saw the Model Act as, in the words of State Representative Melvin Neufeld of Kansas, "just tweaking the system." According to Arvy Smith and Brenda Vossler, in North Dakota the Model Act was used as a means to evaluate current statutes. After significant review and debate regarding quarantine and isolation issues, the North Dakota Legislative Assembly enacted the legislation; but, they continue, "we anticipate further review of our statutes in upcoming sessions."

In Louisiana, says J. Thomas Schedler, the Model Act was accepted virtually intact as the pattern for state legislation; he adds, "We also are going through all of our statutes and executive order policy." The state, he explains, has "a very powerful government by statutes and constitution so a lot of the powers and needs are vested in our governor." The act was useful for the legislators since they were "trying to codify and pull together exactly what we have into one document. It's scattered all over everyplace, and we're trying to match that off with this bill." Schedler believes that "we will find that we have 70 percent of what's in that bill already in place." Missouri, as well, found that it had "incredible powers at the state level already. If the governor declares an emergency," observes Ronald Cates, chief operating officer of the Missouri Department of Health and Senior Services, "he can order anything necessary." From Cates's perspective, the Model Act was useful because it helped the state to "change language" and update the existing law, which had largely been drafted in the nineteenth century when "there was no mention of bioterrorism or terrorism."

Angela Coron, in California, saw no need at all for the Model Act. Because her state had been coping with natural disasters for many years, public health authorities and the legislature "have a lot of experience with this. . . . Public health authorities have legal authority to take action, . . . and the state can direct local authorities to act if they are not taking action." Coron noted that on the day she was interviewed, "a plane from Japan was briefly quarantined because a pilot had concerns about SARS"; even though at the time SARS was not subject to federal quarantine regulations, county health officials in Los Angeles did not hesitate to go "to the plane and take some passengers to the hospital. . . . The whole incident took two hours." Though California law does not address "the broader question about who has the authority to enter the plane and require passengers to go to a hospital," that silence does not prevent public health authorities from acting. Texas as well, according to Dennis Perrotta, has long been prepared for natural disasters, and "the model emergency powers act has been used as a model not to submit to the legislature but to see how we are doing in Texas in terms of policies and actions." The state "did side-by-side comparisons of the Model Act and current Texas statutes to compare capacities and contents," he reports. "We found we were in good shape and only had to do some minor clarifications and updates such as defining what is a public health emergency."

One of the few states that seems to have used the model legislation to make significant changes is Arizona; there, Catherine Eden says, a "core of people within the department [led by David Engelthaler] revised their own laws." If the government declares a bioterrorist emergency, the Department of Health Services is "in the lead," whereas "normally it would be the county." For state officials, "the legislation clarified our role." Less positively, she views the Model Act as trying "to throw in the kitchen sink, but I don't think the legislature or the public were prepared for that. But I think we got a good, decent piece of legislation."

Quarantine

One reason that many state departments of health were ready to accept the Model Act's assertions of state power was their experience over the previous two decades with tuberculosis and HIV/AIDS. Robert Eadie's description of Tennessee as "very aggressive" in dealing with "noncompliant TB patients" to stem the spread of the disease in Nashville and Memphis could apply to many states. And in Tennessee, as noted above, civil libertarians had already been involved in working on regulations to control infectious disease, so new discussions of the state health department's role in dealing with bioterrorism proceeded relatively smoothly.

In Minnesota, in contrast, Lee Greenfield notes that it was very hard "selling the legislature . . . [on] a need to look at quarantine laws." Legislators as well as the general population had forgotten that "these previous epidemics required quarantine. That was history." Greenfield describes the old laws as "very simple": "The commissioner of health had the authority to quarantine, the authority to declare a building a health hazard." But "since everybody in the '80s was saying you can't enforce them anyhow," the legislature removed them. He believes that

we had, might even still have, on the books some remnants of the quarantine laws, but when AIDS broke out in the early 1980s and was being addressed by the states, there was a clear belief that courts would not allow us to use general blanket quarantine laws. In fact, I was the chief author in the Minnesota House of the noncompliant disease carrier bill, which was an alternative, which happens to work for HIV. We were one of the first states that did it — created standards and all — and that was fine, and the whole belief at that time was nobody would get back to quarantine laws. Well, very obviously, if you're going to get a smallpox outbreak or it's a possibility, you need some quarantine, there is no other way to address some things if you don't have a way to treat it. Or the new SARS epidemic. And when it came to the legislature it was just like, "Huh, we don't want to do this." And they barely got a bill through with an agreement that it would be temporary, and we'd have to study it and bring back something next year that'll have to address that.

In Connecticut and Ohio, civil liberties groups more actively opposed the statutes that gave public health authorities the right to quarantine. Their concerns led to Connecticut's "public health emergency law . . . being dissected," in Norma Gyle's words. Similarly, Anne Harnish says that in Ohio, legislators worried about whether "quarantine powers [should] be restricted, which is interesting in light of the SARS epidemic." In Iowa, notes Mary Kramer, there were no major changes in the law, but the "Christian Science community had worked hard to get religious exceptions under our immunization law, and they were concerned about new immunization and quarantine policies. But right now everyone is feeling okay."

In Louisiana the issue of quarantine was "obviously politically charged," according to J. Thomas Schedler. The act was opposed by "the usual suspects" — that is, the ACLU. But, he points out, "this is a very conservative state . . . and the ACLU is usually not successful in most of their projects here. If anything, they're the best people to have against you because if they oppose you, you pretty much know you are going to win." Schedler recognizes that "it sounds horrible — quarantine — but I think most people, if you get them and talk to them, they recognize that that's what has to be done . . . for the betterment of the whole."

Because of its experiences with TB, Arizona's arguments about quarantine were muted; nevertheless, widespread popular antipathy to government intrusion led authorities to scale down those aspects of the Model Act that touched on quarantine. Catherine Eden recalls that "there were things in there like [the] taking of people's property, confiscating weapons, getting onto people's property, which we thought would not be in the purview of public health, which were modified to make them more acceptable. . . . We put in provisions that people can't be forced to be vaccinated [or get] treatment but may be forced, if sick, to be isolated." Interestingly, the state ACLU was fine with the legislation, while conservatives, including those in Phyllis Schlafly's Eagle Forum, "had spent a lot of energy sending things to legislators all across the U.S. saying 'do not sign off.'" Legislators initially made a "big deal" about fighting it, she adds. "But as soon as they saw how reasonable it was . . . most of the conservatives signed off on it, and it went through pretty fast."

Surveillance

Like quarantine, disease surveillance posed civil liberties issues for some state health officials. The Model Act called not only for traditional disease reporting through hospitals and other health centers but also for private physicians and pharmacists to notify state officials of unusual disease patterns, giving specific patient information. Yet little real opposition to these new elements emerged. Most states appear to have been very careful to guard against the release of any personal identifying information, and that care was reinforced by newly implemented provisions of the Health Insurance Portability and Accountability Act of 1996 (HIPAA). Pursuant to the act, in April 2003 the Department of Health and Human Services issued the first federal privacy standards aimed at protecting the medical records and other health information of U.S. citizens, and these new standards raised questions about the ethics of sharing information about communicable diseases with federal authorities. Thus public health professionals discussed key legal and policy matters: What was HIPAA's impact on syndromic surveillance? What "amount of data collected exceeds conventional reporting requirements, [and] has the balance of privacy and public health value been appropriately made?"[137] In Ohio the issue of confidentiality was a concern, especially for some reporters and for the newspapers' association.[138] But despite significant editorial opposition, the Model Act was adopted there in the fall of 2003. Lisa Kaplowitz notes that when the state epidemiologist in Virginia collaborated with Johns Hopkins University to improve disease surveillance, civil libertarians voiced few objections: "Civil libertarians have their hands so full with guns and abortion that there is little time for concern about public health surveillance."

In Kentucky the debate was shaped by an incident in February 2003: state computers with information regarding AIDS patients were "discarded for sale as surplus equipment." One computer, bought for $25 by the state auditor's office, was discovered to contain highly personal — though coded — information. Coming as it did on the heels of widespread attention to the possible civil liberties intrusions of the Model Act, this mishap gained national attention. Kentucky State Auditor Ed Hatchett said that the discarded computers had "a lot of information with lots of names and things like [numbers of] sexual partners of those who are diagnosed with AIDS. . . . It's a terrible security breach."[139] Yet Kentucky's commissioner of public health, Rice Leach, recalls that despite this unfortunate accident, "community trust has been sustained. . . . If you give people all the information, they may not agree with you, but they trust you. I think people trust us." Nor did any protest regarding surveillance emerge in Kansas, North Dakota, Maine, Louisiana, New Jersey, or Texas.[140] As Melvin Neufeld of Kansas comments, "most of the general public did not know or care about what's happening."

Some administrators believed that those who saw the Model Act as radical and possibly undermining of personal liberties by authorizing dramatic intrusions were totally off the mark; to the contrary, they viewed it as a weak political compromise that did not give public health officials the tools they needed to adequately address the threat of bioterrorism or chemical attack. John Chapin had been chastened by his experience with discussion of the Model Act in the Wisconsin State Legislature. "Wisconsin is a classic example of a state with relatively modern public health laws (1993) and strong laws," he observes. "A reasonable set of modifications to the law was proposed." But "it was then thrown into state politics and became a pawn in the partisan budget wars." He worries that the legislature responded not to true public health needs but to irrational fear: "The black helicopter conspiracy believers came out of the woods, the anti-immunization crew joined them, the funeral directors feared the government would seize bodies and their businesses, and state emergency government staff expressed concern because they saw their turf threatened. . . . The result is possibly no legal reform in Wisconsin. . . . In the closing days of the budget debate, it now appears that compromise language has been agreed to, but this just shows how subject to political chance all of this is when left to the states."[141] The legislation was finally enacted in April 2004.

REGIONAL COORDINATION

Perhaps the most glaring weakness highlighted by the events of September 11 and the subsequent anthrax episode was the fragile—indeed, almost nonexistent—relationship between the various state health departments throughout the country. In part, this reflects an exception to one of the major shifts of the twentieth century: the enormous expansion in the scope of federal power and authority, as Washington assumed responsibilities and powers that were once the province of the states. Labor, commerce, environmental regulation, food and drug safety, and a host of other policy concerns have moved from the state and local to the national arena. Yet even as public health is addressed in national agencies such as the Public Health Service and the National Institutes of Health within the Department of Health and Human Services, many critical powers and decisions that affect the nation's health and well-being remain with the states and localities.[142] The practical result has been a striking lack of coordination as states prepare for bioterrorism, with administrators in each state department of health acting in almost total independence. We discuss the centrality of the federal government in these issues in the following chapter.

In late January 2002, in the aftermath of 9/11, State Senator Betty Sims of Missouri called Daniel Fox, president of the Milbank Memorial Fund, to ask if Milbank, on behalf of the Reforming States Group (a nonpartisan organization of senior executives and legislators from the U.S. states and several Canadian provinces), would convene a meeting of officials of states adjacent to Missouri to coordinate their activities. She told Fox that she wanted to bring together legislative leaders, state health officials, and emergency response officials from eight states in addition to her own. This gathering on April 4, 2002, was so successful that Milbank and the Reforming States Group decided to host similar meetings in other regions around the country to focus on the relationships between emergency management personnel, public health officials, and others in government. In the end, seven other meetings were held, drawing in the states surrounding Massachusetts, North Carolina, Texas, Wyoming, Nevada, Maryland, and Wisconsin. Among those attending were emergency management and public health officials, representatives from offices of states' attorneys general, and legislative leaders. The meetings revealed serious misperceptions about the status of readiness among and within the various states. Officials in New England, for example, had been told — erroneously — that coordination was already in place, leading them initially to believe that the exercise was unnecessary. It soon became clear that public health and emergency management personnel rarely talked to each other within, much less across, states. In western states, which had a long experience with natural disasters such as tornadoes, droughts, and fires, coordination was better.

One concrete effort at coordination across state lines was the Emergency Management Assistance Compact (EMAC), described by Washington State's Emergency Management Division as a "mutual aid agreement and partnership between states that exists" to deal with everything "from hurricanes to earthquakes and from wildfires to toxic waste spills or acts of terrorism." The compact was approved by Congress in 1996 because "all states share a common enemy: the constant threat of disaster." By 2003, forty-eight states (all but California and Hawaii) and two territories had passed EMAC-enabling legislation.[143] This legislation creates a mechanism to allow governors to provide assistance to neighboring states without worrying about liability or cost. Initially envisioned for the sharing of personnel and equipment in natural disasters, EMAC was virtually unknown to state public health workers before the meetings sponsored by Milbank and the Reforming States Group. But the threats of anthrax and smallpox pushed public health into the realm of emergency management and made it necessary to adapt the compact to address public health concerns. Issues of liability would now include malpractice, and the personnel moving across state lines would include credentialed medical workers. Who is responsible for the mistakes of a practitioner not licensed to practice in a particular state? What responsibility did one state have to supervise nurses or doctors from other states who traveled to a disaster site?

These efforts have led to some improvements, notably in communicating about and assessing risk. Consider Illinois, for example: if an incident occurs in the southwest corner of the state, it is likely that local television and radio stations will turn to public health officials in neighboring St. Louis for comment and direction, because Missouri media are the major source of local information in southern Illinois. There is a greater recognition of the need for close contact between officials in neighboring media markets. In some states, lawyers are working together to resolve liability and licensing issues that might arise after biological or chemical attacks. The response by the states and federal government to the SARS and monkeypox outbreaks was better than it might have been before 9/11 because of these endeavors. Specifically, officials are cooperating to decide both who should communicate with the public and what their message should be. And John Colmers, program officer of the Milbank Memorial Fund, concludes that surveillance, especially getting and sharing information from hospitals, has improved since 9/11.[144]

Some very practical steps have taken place. In Virginia, reports a magazine published by the Virginia Municipal League, the Department of Health has "coordinated with the Metropolitan Washington Council of

Governments to develop a Regional Incident Communication and Coordination System, as well as related planning." In addition, the "Division of Consolidated Laboratory Services has established a structure to develop and implement a program to provide rapid and effective laboratory services responses to bioterrorism, other infectious disease outbreaks, and other public health threats and emergencies."[145] Louisiana is setting up a training site that could be used by neighboring state emergency and public health workers to prepare for bioterrorist events, Missouri is coordinating with its eight border states to organize cross-border clinics, lawyers in Connecticut are investigating credential and liability issues, and Ohio is negotiating terms for sharing mutual aid assistance and laboratory services with neighboring Indiana.[146] In 2003, the Ohio Department of Health publicized its "contracts with local partners in seven regions to create regional bioterrorism plans."[147] Texas health and emergency management personnel have met with their counterparts in neighboring states at least twice. According to Dennis Perrotta, "public health did not have a long-standing relationship with emergency management, but it does now. For example, the FBI's five agents in charge of weapons of mass destruction now have my home phone number, and I have their cell numbers." Since September 11, "there are plenty of good examples of different agencies working together"; he points to the Columbia shuttle disaster of February 2003 as the most notable.

Some states, it appears, have simply returned to business as usual and continue to work in isolation from their colleagues in other states. In Iowa, for example, notes State Senator Mary Kramer, the interstate compact was passed, and they "are getting licensure agreements approved, so if there is an emergency and, for instance, a registered nurse comes to us from the next state, we know that their qualifications are approved." But there are worries that "the costs of assembling teams are high, and this adds a level of complexity to their jobs." Lee Greenfield observes that in Minnesota, though much of rural Wisconsin is closer to Minneapolis than to Madison, interstate coordination has not progressed very far beyond laws that "tend to recognize emergency staff from one state to the next." To deal with these problems, government officials outside public health agencies will have to apply more pressure.

After conducting a comprehensive survey of states' public health preparedness, the Trust for America's Health published a report in 2003 titled *Ready or Not? Protecting the Public's Health in the Age of Bioterrorism;* it declared that "states are only modestly better prepared to respond to health emergencies than they were prior to September 11, 2001."[148] In testimony in 2004 before the U.S. Congress, Shelley Hearne, the executive director of Trust for America's Health, expressed great concern that "the nation's public health system is being stretched to the breaking point." Although the researchers had found that most states had successfully improved communications and that "every state had at least an initial plan on paper on how to mobilize public health resources in the event of a terrorist attack, they also uncovered "much room for improvement" and "some serious shortcomings." By mid-2004, only three states had achieved "full readiness . . . [w]ith respect to receiving, distributing, and administering emergency vaccinations and antidotes from the Strategic National Stockpile." In addition, "only six states report that they have sufficient laboratory facilities should a major public health emergency occur."[149] In an update of the initial report, completed in December 2004, the Trust for America's Health concluded that "states across the country are still struggling to meet basic preparedness requirements and have inadequate resources to juggle the competing health priorities they face." Despite "incremental progress," the Trust found that "many basic bioterrorism detection, diagnosis, and response capabilities are still not in place."[150] A 2005 report by the Council of State and Territorial Epidemiologists similarly noted that although "increased funding . . . has rapidly increased the number of epidemiologists and increased capacity for preparedness at the state level," 45.3 percent more would be "needed nationwide to fully staff terrorism preparedness programs."[151] These reports indicate that while the states need to make bioterrorism preparedness and building up the public health infrastructure a higher priority, the responsibility for providing guidance and funds to achieve those ends rests mainly with the federal government.[152]

THREE

EMERGENCY PREPAREDNESS, BIOTERRORISM, AND THE CDC

Federal Involvement before and after 9/11

Public health activities have traditionally been understood as state and local functions. Throughout the nineteenth and twentieth centuries, disease surveillance and reporting, quarantine, vaccination campaigns, and treatment — as well as sanitation and other preventive strategies — were carried out largely by local and state health departments. The Centers for Disease Control and Prevention (CDC) has steadily grown into the preeminent federal health authority, but it has always provided advice and support at the local level, not taken command. In the days after the attacks of 9/11, however, federal staff and resources quickly became more directly involved in what was clearly a national emergency — and particularly in New York, some aspects of the relationship between the local and federal health authorities became more problematic.

Richard Jackson, former director of the National Center for Environmental Health of the CDC, notes that CDC staff were sent to New York City to help with a variety of tasks, including routine data collection that the city was unable to perform, because the CDC was "very worried that there might be some other kind of biological or chemical event going on."[1] He recalls,

> We were doing just a lot of tracking in emergency rooms, and reporting up, because everyone wanted to know, "What is the morbidity? Who's been hurt? What are the numbers? Is it getting better? Is it getting worse? What sort of respiratory disease problems are we seeing?" . . . So we were tracking for anything that looked odd or peculiar coming into the emergency rooms

with the rest. It was very interesting in emergency rooms, because at first we were getting a lot of resistance from the docs — not from the nurses or the administrative staff, but the physicians in emergency rooms were like, "Why are these epidemiologists, these kids," because they were mostly twenty-eight-year-old young physicians, "running around and asking questions of everybody that's coming in." . . . While the initial response was extraordinary, problems in communication, lines of authority, and control quickly led to differences and conflict. . . . Particularly when an emergency would come in, and they'd bypass Admitting and go directly to a code room, code blue room, we'd have our young folks sort of hovering over them, trying to find out what was going on. We were getting a fair amount of resistance. Honestly, it wasn't till anthrax appeared — and we had told them, "Don't say why you're doing this, because we don't want to spread alarm." It wasn't till anthrax raised its head — suddenly the docs who were obstructing us, it suddenly dawned on them why we were bird-dogging these cases so closely.

Jeffrey Koplan, then the director of the CDC, believes that despite some minor irritations, his agency's relationship with local health officials on the ground after 9/11 was generally good because procedures between the CDC and the state and local authorities had already been worked out. He explains, "In public health events of great or minor scope the standard operating procedure is that if the event is in one state, the personnel in that state are in charge. If that state calls in help from the CDC we send staff to help but the state is in charge." As the dimensions of the attack became clear, the CDC maintained this tradition: the epidemiologists who were sent to New York "were always subservient to the New York [City] personnel." The CDC had found over time, says Koplan, "that the system doesn't work well if the feds show up and take over."[2] On the other hand, as Jackson points out, it was important for federal officials to anticipate the needs of local officials. He remembers what happened when he had to deal with disasters in California:

One of the things I learned after the riots and the fires and the rest is I would call, for example, the Los Angeles Health Department: "Do you need any help?" "No, we're fine. We're okay." You'd call the next day. "Do you need any help? Do you want me to send anybody?" "No. We're fine." I'd call the third day. "Damn it! Why the hell didn't you send somebody? We're dying down here. We're working twenty-four hours a day, and our families are yelling for us," because they have their own sets of problems with the earthquake or whatever it is. So the lesson I learned is even if the locality says, "We're fine. Don't send help," send help up, because if nothing else they can do the routine stuff, whether it's rat bites or something else, they can do the routine stuff when folks are just getting overwhelmed with other problems.

The CDC found a compatible partner in the New York City Department of Health. "Neal Cohen was the commissioner of health and we worked well with him," Koplan recalls. When Jackson and Koplan arrived in the city on October 3 they met with Cohen, to discuss disease surveillance and other issues. Jackson says, "We visited ground zero, and it was—I'm a good talker, as you can tell from this tape, or can be long-winded. Dr. Koplan is a wonderful talker, and there wasn't a word said for fifteen minutes as we went around the site. It was just—we were dumbstruck by the magnitude of the World Trade Center event. Even then, the smells and the dust in the air, three or four weeks later—it was tremendous."

The CDC officials then visited the mayor's newly established operations center at Pier 92, "where there were forty agencies represented around a large table, reporting on everything ranging from alternate side of the street parking to mortician issues to social service issues and the rest. I have to tell you, it was inspiring to see how tightly and effectively that was run. There was no really silly banter. It was . . . very, very impressive. . . . I've worked with political leaders long enough to become as cynical as anyone, and there was nothing to be cynical about. This was taken with such seriousness." Koplan and Jackson toured the pier; ten CDC employees were already at work. Jackson continues, "It was really inspiring, because there were probably 1,000 people there. . . . I met with Mr. Gabriel, who was the head of emergency medical services. . . . He described his having to evacuate the command center at the Trade Center, and his experiences, and how when they arrived at Pier 92 to establish a whole new center, that the cellular companies, the wireless companies, the computer companies, arrived. Without any discussion, no discussion of contracts or anything else—even now it sort of brings tears to my eyes—just the whole place was set up in about six to eight hours."

Jackson recalls that "there were computer systems and there were large screen TVs and they were tracking what was going on. At this table there were the CDC people, and then there was the state health department, and then there was EPA [the Environmental Protection Agency], and then there was the Coast Guard, and then there was the FBI, and then there was the military, and one security agency after another. People were walking back and forth, and there was such—never in my whole career had I ever experienced such a sense of superb management and seamless coordination around a series of important issues. It could not have functioned more effectively. I never had seen anything look so seamless." Jackson acknowledges that "probably behind the circle there was still interagency shoving and the rest, but nothing compared to what you would see like in Washington or anywhere else, in a non-catastrophic episode."

Of particular interest to Jackson were the psychological issues.

> We set up a team to work with the city health department to do a survey at four different strata of populations, going out from ground zero, both people who were geographically impacted as well as people who were personally impacted, whether it was the loss of a loved one or a coworker or something else. . . . We developed a questionnaire that was derived from one that was used at the Pentagon around post-traumatic stress syndrome, looking at what were you doing, what sort of behaviors do you do to modify some of the stresses you're under. We're very interested in what's the best way to handle the psychological trauma that people were going through. That data is now being analyzed as well.

He "assigned two people over time up [in New York]. One was my deputy for all of policy, a very senior fellow named Michael Sage. Mike is a very good manager, a very good person in communications and policy. I put him up here for a couple of weeks," because "Mike was very good at just how you think about the structure and the organization, and how you move people, and how you maximize. One of the things in emergencies is a lot of times people don't pace themselves, and they deplete rapidly." After a couple of weeks, "the head of environmental health services — a physician named Pat Meehan — came up, and both of them were either at the health officer's elbow or at the mayor's elbow during much of this time."

The other senior CDC official in New York was Stephen Ostroff, at the time the associate director for epidemiologic science at the National Center for Infectious Diseases. Ostroff, who later became deputy director of NCID, recalls that he "was not technically the leader of the CDC effort in NYC"; but since the "other CDC officers were not Infectious Disease people" he emerged as a central federal official in New York. There were two groups of federal disease specialists in New York. The first were Epidemic Intelligence Service (EIS) officers who "were placed in health care facilities to track individuals affected and spot changing patterns in the hospitals themselves. They collected data." Ostroff "wasn't involved in that but . . . helped facilitate their activities." In the other group were occupational health responders from the National Institute for Occupational Safety and Health and the National Center for Environmental Health.

ANTHRAX

In October, Americans discovered that anthrax had been sent through the mail. After a letter containing the bacteria was opened in the America Media building in Boca Raton, Florida, three people were infected; one died. Koplan recalls, "For the first few days, Florida was in control. . . . All press releases were issued jointly by Florida and the CDC." If the CDC started saying things on its own, "it would have undermined the state officials."

Soon thereafter Tom Brokaw at NBC News also received an anthrax-contaminated letter, and Brokaw's assistant developed a cutaneous form of the disease. Both these letters had been postmarked at a post office in Trenton, New Jersey, and workers there were tested for anthrax exposure. Barely two weeks later, staff and aides to Senators Tom Daschle and Russ Feingold tested positive for exposure to anthrax after another anthrax-contaminated letter was opened on October 15. According to one contemporary report, between October 4 and November 7, the CDC "confirmed a total of 10 cases of inhalational anthrax and 7 cases of cutaneous anthrax. . . . All but 1 of these cases appears to have been directly linked to the US postal system."[3] (It later became clear that in all, there were eleven cases of cutaneous and eleven of inhalation anthrax; two could not be directly linked to the post.)[4] The anthrax episode marked another important and taxing moment in the evolving relationship between the federal and local authorities. Koplan explains,

> As anthrax unfolded with the first case in New York it was no longer an isolated event and this was a major shift. We sent out teams to every site where new cases or problems arose. And there were backup teams in Atlanta that *just* communicated with that team. There was a marked realignment of personnel. One hundred people were pulled from other programs to work on anthrax and even though other programs were sacrificed I'd do it again in a minute. An emergency operations center was set up on Friday and I met with the heads of the different centers and I said we need your *best* people. On Saturday morning they started coming in and they were the best people from all over the CDC.

Ostroff recalls that he "went to New York on the Friday after the first case on Thursday night, around the 12th or the 13th . . . to support the city health department. I had had extended experience with the New York City Department of Health because of the West Nile episodes in 1999 and 2000. I knew the health commissioner, I had been involved in press conferences with the health commissioner and the deputy mayor regarding West Nile. Since I had experience I became involved with media issues. I went to help direct communications, not so much the scientific matters, but to help handle media and coordination issues." After anthrax was discovered in Washington D.C.'s Brentwood facility (two of whose workers died), the CDC

> offered prophylaxis to everyone at the Morgan facility [the main mail sorting and distribution center in Manhattan]; but when the CDC representatives spoke to city officials, they said it was a federal facility and not a city problem. They didn't completely wash their hands of it since the victims were residents of New York City, and they did provide communication and personnel, but by and large, the intervention was from the federal level. We mobilized the public health service people in twenty-four hours to get antibiotics to NYC. We didn't have a plan at that point but we coordinated with the postal service itself. It was amazing at how the effort was carried out out of camera range. There are tunnels in and out of the facility and we got the antibiotics distributed in twenty-four hours without the press knowing.

Ostroff stayed in New York "for two weeks and then went home on a Friday for the weekend." But "the following Monday was when the Vietnamese woman [Kathy Nguyen, who later died] came down with anthrax. When I left, there was concern about my leaving, . . . but I said that I would return if there was any other incident. So I returned that Monday." The demands on his time grew immensely as anthrax cases appeared in other localities. "I had been asked to go to Trenton to help with the postal service and to participate in a press conference. I was supposed to go to Washington, D.C., on Tuesday for a congressional hearing but changed plans on Tuesday morning. . . . I came back to New York a third time to testify in a lawsuit brought by the postal union against the postal service."

It was clear to Ostroff that he

> had never experienced anything so intense. Everything was intense. There were continual demands, constant issues and problems that needed to be handled on a day to day basis. The anthrax letters, the onslaughts of meetings, issues that were arising continuously, there just wasn't enough time. The fact that it came on the heels of September 11 made it just unique, made it intense. People were so worn out, so tired by 9/11 and then to overlay anthrax on top of all of this brought people to the breaking point. No one knew what was coming next. There were unending demands — people there rose to the challenge but they could only maintain themselves so long before reaching a breaking point. It was the torrent of calls, high pressure situations, press conferences with the mayor, and preparations for them

early in the morning, dealing with the mayor's advisory group in the afternoon. The pressure was constant.

At every turn, he found unexpected new demands. "Some issues seemed simple, such as how to get from point A to point B," Ostroff remembers. But even his own movements became complex: "Areas of the city were closed off but I needed to be at meetings and I was caught in traffic jams." One time he "did a national interview with NPR on a cell phone and fading in and out between buildings." Every day he would start out doing one or two morning shows. "One morning I did all three of them, then found myself racing to city hall for the mayor's meeting. By nine o'clock I was wrung out. I had no time to eat or sleep. Even communicating with my office in Atlanta was a problem. I had to have a person dealing with the phone calls and scheduling for me. Certain days I was worried about my health, I was worried about collapsing at the mayor's press conference and that would be embarrassing."

Unprecedented demands were also made on the CDC's technical and scientific expertise and facilities, further stressing the already highly taxed agency. "We needed epidemiologists, people with shoes on the ground," Ostroff recalls. "At the peak we had thirty to forty assisting the various aspects of the investigation as part of our response." Even the relatively sophisticated and extensive facilities of the New York City Department of Health were overwhelmed: "There were very significant challenges with the laboratories. They were very overstretched by September 11 and they were getting absolutely deluged with [suspected anthrax] specimens to test. There were rooms filled with specimens from public health department officials, stacks and stacks of letters to process, even a mirror someone sent in with some dust on it. There was not even a system for prioritizing these samples." James Hughes, director of the National Center for Infectious Diseases, suggests that the "middle tier of state and federal labs was overwhelmed even though there were a limited number of cases on the East Coast. The network processed tens of thousands of specimens."[5]

One incident stood out for Ostroff as exemplifying the problems facing the public health community: "the NBC letter contaminated the testing suite. The policeman came in and was himself contaminated and the facility had to shut down." Ed Thompson, then the chief of public health improvement in the CDC's Office of the Director, observes that even though the focus was on the few states where anthrax exposures had been verified, the entire public health system was put to the test. "At the time of the anthrax attack everyone spoke about the five states that were directly affected, but the other forty-five states had to test hundreds of samples and rule them out, and as a result of the CDC's training we were able to do that without having to send them to the CDC. As a result," Thompson concludes, "we were able to reassure individuals and keep businesses operating" despite the massive strains on the nation's laboratories. Thompson believes that "the most important part of the federal response to the anthrax attacks occurred prior to the event. The CDC trained state labs to identify anthrax and other Category A agents [i.e., those seen as posing the greatest potential threat to public health, with a moderate to high potential for large-scale dissemination]. Before that they would have to send all the samples to Atlanta."[6]

Stephen Ostroff acknowledges some other problems as well. "Risk communication was not handled well—I said some things in public and private that I regret having said. I was reacting based on what I considered dogma that turned out to be incorrect, like who needed prophylaxis and who didn't and what were the risks to workers. Remember the hullabaloo about nasal swabs, and challenges around decontamination were major lapses and gaps. It was a no-win situation, but it could have been done better." Complicating the CDC's work was intense political pressure to produce accurate data quickly. "There were tremendous demands from those who wanted results in real time," recalls Ostroff. "We brought in resources and the Department of Defense brought in a whole emergency lab." Furthermore, the existing administrative structures prevented efficient management of the crisis. He explains,

> One of the major problems we faced was that we had to report to many different heads and there were too many demands, from the White House, Congress, the mayor, the HHS [Department of Health and Human Services], our own people at the CDC, everyone. There were too many cooks. And everyone had to know first. It was an enormous challenge to help with both the communication and the scientific aspects. Everyone wanted to be the first to know the most minor scintilla of information — the White House, Congress, the mayor, the city's health department, the state; and there were the most important people, the victims — the networks, the postal service, as well as the literal victims, those who were sick. The problem was that as soon as you gave one piece of information then it was out immediately. The networks were victims so as soon as information was given to them, the CDC, the White House, and everyone was upset that they hadn't been informed first. The person who was most upset was the mayor.

Jeffrey Koplan felt these pressures in Atlanta: "After September 11 we were sending folks up to New York and the White House issued a communications edict whereby all information flows from there, which was fine. And for several weeks all information was cleared first with HHS and the city." But, he recalls, dealing with the public fears of anthrax raised the strain on federal officials to a new level. "When anthrax cases showed up in New York, the White House and HHS became heavily involved"; as a result, Koplan says, conflicts began to emerge between the CDC and HHS: "The CDC asked if they could make general responses to questions and I asked if I could go on *60 Minutes*." He explored this possibility with HHS and the White House and was "given brackets about what I was allowed to say. . . . In the end I refused to do it. Instead, Secretary Thompson appeared on the show. HHS was perfectly within its purview and it wanted more control over its agencies. And I didn't mind that. They wanted more control to be exercised by Washington. And they perceived that I was resistant to that level of control." Because Secretary Thompson and the Bush administration had only recently come into office, the various administrators had no preexisting relationships. Without that personal comfort level, the administration became "anxious about not being kept in the loop. In this kind of a crisis you can guarantee that all parties will not be as well-informed as they want to be."

Inside-the-Beltway politics amplified the tensions between the CDC in Atlanta and the Bush administration. "In Washington, D.C.," Koplan points out, "everyone thinks they are in charge—the chief health people for the House and the Senate, elected officials, HHS, local health authorities—each says, 'I'm important here.' If you look at any of the news reports, usually local health officials step forward first and then when the questions become more difficult, they would bring in the CDC people to answer them."

Joseph Henderson, then chief of program operations for bioterrorism preparedness and response at the Centers for Disease Control and now CDC senior management official to the New York State Department of Health, blames the agency's problems partly on long-standing organizational weaknesses. The CDC "never had a system of command and control before anthrax," he argues. "They did not have the training to deal with a crisis of this magnitude and complexity. They could only react. On a daily basis situation briefings were held for Dr. Koplan and the CDC leadership. Too often there would be standing room only in the CDC director's conference room trying to provide updates on CDC response and as a result decision making became difficult and confused." Henderson believes that the CDC had "done a fantastic job collecting data and information to support decision making, but the rapid speed in having to analyze the data challenged CDC's scientists, who were not comfortable working under these pressures to produce conclusions. Therefore decision making, both tactical and strategic, was not in concert and was often slow relative to the rapidly escalating public health emergency. CDC was also handicapped by not being able to work openly with the media relative to CDC response activities." In his view, the agency was helped greatly by Julie Gerberding, then serving as acting deputy director of NCID, who "was able to coordinate our thinking and brought us out of that funk. She was the one who had the steady hand and this led to her being named to the head of the CDC. But the basic problem was that the agency was not configured to these kinds of things. But under Dr. G. it is now able to do so because strategic and tactical issues are separated."[7]

Anthrax continued to haunt federal officials long after the initial attacks. In an interview in mid-2004, Stephen Ostroff said that he continued "to have a profound sense of sadness that all of this has happened in the first place. It really troubles me that we haven't gotten the perpetrator of the anthrax event yet and that is really frightening." Shortly after the mailings he was asked if he thought the perpetrator would be found and he answered that he certainly thought so, adding, "I won't sleep well until he is found." A few weeks later, a newspaper person asked him, "How are you sleeping?"

FROM EMERGENCY RESPONSE TO TERRORISM AND BIOTERRORISM

In the decade before the attacks of September 11, the federal government had come to terms with the possibility and the reality of terrorism as a fact of life in America. Before the 1990s, it had a relatively limited role in emergency preparedness. Under the Robert T. Stafford Disaster Relief and Emergency Act of 1974, the president could declare federal emergencies and was authorized to develop a federal response plan. Although the Federal Emergency Management Agency (FEMA) was established in 1979 to coordinate federal disaster responses, it did not promulgate any federal response plan until 1992. As amended in 1999 and 2000, that plan represented an agreement between twenty-seven federal agencies and the American Red Cross to provide local, state, and federal agencies with guidance in the event of a terrorist attack in the United States.[8]

The federal response to public health emergencies has a much longer history, rooted in distinct roles for local health authorities and for federal agencies concerned with keeping disease from crossing our borders and protecting our military personnel overseas. Protecting the health of sailors was among the first federal responsibilities recognized, as the U.S. Marine Hospital Service was established in 1798. But not until 1878 did the National Quarantine Act of 1878 transfer authority to impose quarantines from the states to the Marine Hospital Service, reorganized as the U.S. Public Health Service in 1912. Throughout the nineteenth and twentieth centuries, various federal agencies and departments had overlapping and sometimes conflicting roles in emergency preparedness. The Communicable Disease Center, later expanded and renamed as the Centers for Disease Control and Prevention, was established in 1946; the current Department of Health and Human Services, previously the Department of Health, Education and Welfare, houses the Office of Public Health Preparedness that was established in November 2001.[9]

The Marine Hospital Service and the U.S. Public Health Service, in its early decades, focused on keeping people with infectious diseases out of the United States by carrying out inspections (and, when necessary, quarantines) of immigrants and commercial shipping and, later, by conducting research into tropical diseases that threatened American military forces in Central America, the Caribbean, and the Philippines. Similarly, the CDC concentrated first on infectious diseases (initially malaria) and subsequently expanded its scope to chronic diseases and other health threats. In the second half of the twentieth century, the line between traditional local health department activities and those carried out by the federal agencies became less clear. As global health problems such as AIDS, monkeypox, SARS (severe acute respiratory syndrome), and other infectious diseases grew in importance in the 1990s, so did federal involvement in local and state health activities. Bioterrorism brought into high relief the need to address the changing relationships between the federal and state health authorities.

Other events in the 1990s highlighted U.S. vulnerabilities and focused the government's attention; James Hughes points to a report in 1992 by the Institute of Medicine on emerging infectious microbial diseases threatening the country; outbreaks of E. coli O157:H7 in 1992 and 1993; a mysterious, severe respiratory illness (now known as hantavirus pulmonary syndrome) on a Navaho reservation in Arizona in 1993; and the emergence of Ebola virus in Zaire (now the Democratic Republic of the Congo) in 1995. That last would prove to be a critical year in the evolution of America's understanding of the international and national dimensions of terrorism and bioterrorism as part of our emergency response planning. The bombing of the Alfred P. Murrah Federal

Building in Oklahoma City, the use of chemical agents — sarin gas — in the Japanese subway system by the Aum Shinrikyo cult, and the defection of Saddam Hussein's son-in-law Lieutenant General Hussein Kamel Hassan, who revealed the existence of an Iraqi bioweapons program, combined in 1995 to mobilize the federal government. In June, President Clinton issued Presidential Decision Directive 39, a classified directive that named the Department of Health and Human Services and the Veterans Administration as the agencies responsible for stockpiling pharmaceuticals, antidotes, and vaccines and also for training medical responders in the National Disaster Medical Systems hospitals.

In 1996, federal efforts to prepare for unexpected terrorist attacks expanded. The Presidential Commission on Critical Infrastructure Protection set forth a national strategy to protect the nation from physical and computer threats. Also in 1996 Congress passed the Defense against Weapons of Mass Destruction Act (P.L. 104-201), which established a domestic preparedness program that provided training, expertise, and grants for equipment to 120 cities; created the chemical and biological response team within the Department of Defense; and directed the Department of Health and Human Services to form metropolitan medical response teams in the nation's largest metropolitan areas. The act also directed FEMA, which had previously focused on natural disasters such as hurricanes, fires, landslides, and earthquakes, both to integrate responses to weapons of mass destruction into its federal response plan and to develop a rapid response system.[10]

In the mid-1990s Ed Thompson, then with the Mississippi Health Department, was on the Executive Committee of the Association of State and Territorial Health Officials (ASTHO). He recalls that a few state officials in the organization "were worried about our ability to respond to or even detect a Category A agent that was let loose on the population." They were especially concerned about smallpox and the lack of sufficient vaccine to address the threat, and he then "testified before Congress on behalf of ASTHO that we needed to get more resources and to spend them wisely."

In fiscal year 1997, the federal government spent about $6.7 billion on terrorism and bioterrorism preparedness. But because the General Accounting Office (the GAO, now the Government Accountability Office) found it impossible to determine precisely how that money was spent, the National Defense Authorization Act of the following year required the Office of Management and Budget to develop a system for collecting and reporting on bioterrorism. Also in 1998, a presidential decision directive created a new position: the national coordinator for security, infrastructure protection, and counterterrorism would be responsible for integrating all government policies and programs that addressed terrorist threats at home and abroad. A key initiative related to bioterrorism was the CDC's establishment of the Bioterrorism Preparedness and Response Program, which focused on five areas: (1) preparedness planning and response, (2) epidemiology and surveillance, (3) biological laboratory capacity, (4) chemical laboratory capacity, and (5) health communications, including the Health Alert Network to bolster public health communications on the state and local levels. In addition, it set up a laboratory response network linking public health departments to improve diagnostic capabilities. In 1998, Congress passed the Omnibus Consolidated and Emergency Supplemental Appropriations Act, which authorized giving $51 million to the CDC to establish a store of pharmaceuticals and vaccines (the National Pharmaceutical Stockpile, later renamed the Strategic National Stockpile).[11] Jeffrey Koplan argues that Congress acted in part because of the CDC's own increased awareness of the threat of bioterrorism: "It started in 1998. In the summer of 1997, I met with the Center directors, and Jim Hughes of Infectious Diseases said, 'It's not a case of if, but when. And it is likely to be during the time you are here.' So, it was on our radar screen and we started beefing up our capabilities." Previously, the CDC had minimal "investment in areas like anthrax; . . . in early 1998 it began to reestablish labs with expert capabilities. It established a rapid response, analysis, and testing lab [RRAT] and put in place a triage lab from which samples were sent out after an initial evaluation."

Joseph Henderson remembers that before 1999, "the CDC didn't receive money to support bioterrorism response. As a result, capacities were not in place nationally nor at CDC to address needed laboratory diagnostic testing for anthrax, smallpox, and plague, nor were disease surveillance systems to detect an outbreak as sensitive as was needed to discover a bioterrorism event, and public health and traditional emergency responders were not trained and equipped to work together in a response to protect the nation's health." He believes that

> the public health system had been in crisis for a couple of decades. For example, it was unprepared for the measles outbreak in the late 1980s. Much of this changed with the infusion of federal dollars to support public health emergency preparedness. In 1999, CDC first established a bioterrorism preparedness and response program office within the National Center for Infectious Diseases. Approximately $120 million was available that first

year to begin to develop or redevelop response capabilities at CDC and at the state and local levels of the public health system. Prior to 9/11, CDC was managing a bioterrorism preparedness and response budget of $189 million, of which $50 million was supporting state and local capacities. In the months following 9/11 this appropriation grew to $2.3 billion with $1 billion going to support state and local response efforts.

Scott Lillibridge, currently professor of epidemiology and director of the Center for Biosecurity and Public Health Preparedness at the University of Texas Health Science Center, recalls his experiences as the first director of the Bioterrorism and Response Program within NCID in 1998. He felt that "no one else at the CDC shared [his] vision or cared" as much as he did about bioterrorism. He was particularly sensitive to the issue because during the mid-1990s he repeatedly came face-to-face with terrorism and bioterrorism. He had been the lead physician during the United States Public Health Service response to the Oklahoma City bombing, he had led the U.S. medical delegation to Japan after the Aum Shinrikyo sect had released sarin in the Tokyo subway, and in 1996 he had served as the Department of Health and Human Services science advisor to the Task Force for Biological and Chemical Terrorist Prevention. He was also the CDC team leader in Denver in 2000 for TOPOFF 1,[12] the first of the exercises involving top government officials (hence the name) that simulated a response to terrorist attacks involving weapons of mass destruction. Congress had passed legislation mandating such simulations in 1998, following the sarin attacks in the Tokyo subway. TOPOFF 1 was conducted under the auspices of the Department of Justice and FEMA.

Initially, Lillibridge recalls, the "threat of bioterrorism was seen as minimal and the prevailing view was 'get a real job.' It was not until 9/11 that the issue caught on." Unlike Koplan and others, Lillibridge sharply criticizes the CDC's actions in the late 1990s; before September 11, he says, "the CDC flatlined our budget to make room for other priorities. At that time the budget was $3.5 billion and now it is $7.1 billion. All the growth is in preparedness dollars. . . . After September 11 everyone became an expert and everyone became a champion of preparedness." He believes that even the efforts that were made in bioterrorism were fragmented because the CDC felt it had to "feed all the constituents," and he declares: "Training was separated, stockpiling was separate. Imagine, I was in charge of bioterrorism preparedness and these areas were outside of my control."

Federal funding for counterterrorism increased from $6.5 billion in

FY 1998 to about $10 billion for FY 2000; HHS's budget for bioterrorism initiatives increased from $14 million to $230 million in FY 2000. According to Koplan, "After 1999 we realized that our building and facilities were grossly inadequate to deal with a national event. We went to Congress and met with Congressman [John] Porter on the Appropriations Committee to add additional funds for full funding for their building campaign for a lab which was only half the size of what we needed. And that was the lab that was used in the evaluation of the anthrax attack. Beginning in 2000 we made funding requests every year but they were not listened to." James Hughes remembers "an infusion of resources for BT preparedness really beginning in 1999. That was when we organized the laboratory response network, which was initially focused on biologic threats but also played a role in addressing chemical threats. There was a dramatic increase in the budget. Of course it was concerned with biological and radiological threats. They took the threat of BT seriously. They have always been trying to increase capacity for tracking infectious diseases and biological threats through dual utility of resources."

In 1999 President Clinton proposed a FY 2000 budget that allocated $10 billion for defense against terrorism and weapons of mass destruction. That figure included $43.4 million (a 150 percent increase over the previous year's allocation) for HHS to address bioterrorism, as well as other money allocated to the National Institutes of Health and the Food and Drug Administration for, among other activities, genetic research and the development of vaccines and drugs. Appropriations for the Metropolitan Medical Response Systems and for improved national, state, and local laboratories were intended to build up the public health infrastructure.[13] Also in 1999, Jeffrey Koplan, the head of the CDC, held a meeting to develop a plan for stockpiling smallpox vaccine; among those attending were officials from the Pentagon, FDA, NIH, and HHS. In an article published in the *New Yorker,* Richard Preston described the scene: "Some two dozen officials flew to Atlanta and gathered around a long table in a room near Koplan's office. One participant, who took notes, said that after the door was closed, Jeff Koplan made it clear — very calmly and politely — that no one would be allowed to leave the room until there was a plan for creating an adequate stockpile of smallpox vaccine. 'I want to know the plan for next week and for next month. I want to see timetables. When are you going to get this done?' he said." As Preston pointed out, Koplan was one of a very small group of doctors anywhere in the world who had actually treated patients who were dying of smallpox:

Koplan encountered smallpox in 1973. He had just finished his medical residency and joined the CDC as an officer in the Epidemic Intelligence Service. He was sent to Bangladesh during the world's last outbreaks of *Variola major*. . . . He set up a ward in the infectious disease hospital in Dacca. . . . He learned how to diagnose smallpox with his fingertips. "A blind person can diagnose smallpox from the feel of the lesions," he says. "Smallpox lesions have a velvety feel. While they look like bubbles on the top of the skin, they feel much more deep-seated." Koplan found nothing he did could change the outcome of the disease. Twenty-six years later, he did not want to have to manage an outbreak of smallpox in the American population.[14]

Jackson notes that "the size of the effort to create the entire Strategic National Stockpile was enormous for CDC," and they were under "a lot of pressure . . . to put this within the Department of Defense, but it turned out the Department of Defense is very good at responding to their own sets of emergencies, but in a civilian episode, it was much smarter for us to work with the drug industry. We had to design our own crates that would go on and off the plane — you know, the containers that you see being loaded on the plane." He explains the complexity of the operation: the CDC

> contracted with two of the biggest air freight companies. We designed mobile containers that would be moved on and off the planes. We constructed eight push packages that were located around the United States. A push package is all presealed, pre-shrink-wrapped, palletized, and in-the-container material that could be flown or moved anywhere in the United States within eight to ten hours. . . . One push package sounds like it's small. In fact, I had envisioned a couple of pallets, shrink-wrapped. It's two 747s worth of material. The quantity of material is enormous. I did not know there was a specialty called "logistician." We ended up hiring a half-dozen logisticians from the military. There are software programs that tell you precisely how to load every single container, how you bar code every little box in there, how you make sure you know which box has the Cipro, which one has the ventilator, which one has the atropine and the rest.

Transporting such huge amounts of material required practice; in a drill in August 2001, Jackson says, "We actually moved this from one site to another. The air freight companies have 747s ready for us, round the clock. They have them around the clock for their own needs as well, but they have agreed that they will load this" — and hundreds of thousands of individual items, all of which had to be identifiable to authorities at faraway locations, were ready to move "within an hour." The skills of the shipping companies were invaluable, he notes: "They were so much more efficient in moving this kind of stuff — loading and moving materiel — than anything the Department of Defense could do, because they're moving tanks or Humvees. It's a totally different drill, and private industry is very good at moving stuff efficiently. I mean, they live or die on their ability to deliver stuff in the morning. So that partnership worked very well. We don't pay a nickel for their being at the ready. It's a couple hundred thousand if we use one of the those planes, but when the time comes, you use it."

Jackson points out that dealing with the drugs was even more complex, because the CDC had to have

> about eight times as much material in vendor-managed inventory. One of the things about buying drugs is you don't really want to buy them. They expire in a year or two or three. Cipro, you know, a hundred bucks a course or so, you don't want to be buying things that are going to be expiring in a year or two. So the next thing the logisticians did was develop a rotational method, where the stuff was moved in. You kept it in stock, and then six or eight months before expiration date, it was then moved in the channels of trade. Once they get to the hospitals with this, it's used very, very rapidly. It's gone. We're very proud of the fact — we've never allowed a single product in the stockpile to expire. We've always moved it through. So in a sense, we're almost leasing the material even though we theoretically own it. The other thing we do with the vendor-managed inventory is the big drug companies have an entire wall that has CDC posters on it, and stuff is sent over there and kept for a period of time.

In May 2000 the Department of Justice, as mandated by Congress, conducted the first TOPOFF exercise for bioterrorism preparedness. It simulated three simultaneous bioterrorism attacks: a pneumonic plague epidemic in Denver, Colorado; the release of a chemical agent in Portsmouth, New Hampshire; and the explosion of a radiological dispersal device near Washington, D.C.[15] The exercise helped federal officials see the many deficiencies in their preparations: no coordination at the state and local levels, no local bioterrorism plans, too few health care workers to deal with a crisis, too few hospital beds for the injured, and inadequate stockpiles of drugs and other needed supplies. At the time, some critics believed that exercises like TOPOFF "focused disproportionately on the on-scene sirens and rescue components of unconventional terrorism response." What was missing, they argued, was basic public health support: "only about 6 percent of the unconventional terrorism budget was devoted to strengthening the public health infrastructure in 2000, but multiple benefits will result because more laboratories can identify infrequently seen diseases and communications within the health care community will be improved."[16]

In November 2000, Congress passed and President Clinton signed the Public Health Improvement Act; some parts of this comprehensive public health package addressed traditional concerns, such as research on lupus and prostate cancer, while others dealt with the response to terrorism and bioterrorism. One component, which had been initially introduced by Senator Bill Frist, sought to strengthen "the nation's capacity to detect and respond to serious public health threats, including antimicrobial resistance and bioterrorist attacks." The act also established a public health emergency fund and authorized $180 million to the CDC for the construction of new facilities and renovation of existing facilities. Moreover, it directed the Secretary of HHS, "in coordination with the Secretary of Defense, to establish a joint interdepartmental working group on preparedness and readiness on the medical and public health effects of a bioterrorist attack on the civilian population. A further working group is established in coordination with FEMA, 'Public Health and Medical Consequences of Bioterrorism.'"[17]

In June 2001, the "Dark Winter" exercise took place. Like TOPOFF, it gave the federal government the opportunity — rare since the civil defense drills of the 1950s — to evaluate its ability to intervene quickly and effectively at the local level. But, analysts point out, Dark Winter was unlike TOPOFF in that it "was a *tabletop* senior level exercise" (rather than a simulation in the field). It was not "a federally conducted exercise, but was created by non-governmental organizations (NGOs) and educational institutions[:] . . . the Johns Hopkins Center for Civilian Biodefense Studies, the Center for Strategic and International Studies, the Analytic Services (ANSER) Institute for Homeland Security, and the Oklahoma Institute for the Prevention of Terrorism." The exercise "simulated an attack on the United States involving the simultaneous release of weaponized smallpox in three different shopping malls in Oklahoma City, Oklahoma, Philadelphia, Pennsylvania, and Atlanta, Georgia."[18] According to Scott Lillibridge, Dark Winter illustrated a number of areas that needed improvement. First was "rapid diagnosis" of biological agents, which "will require strong linkages between clinical and public health laboratories." Second was the "targeting of limited smallpox vaccine stocks to ensure strategic use of vaccine for persons at highest risk of infection." Third was "maintaining effective communications with the media and press during such an emergency," because "the need for accurate and timely information during a crisis is paramount to maintaining the trust of the community." And the final point was providing "early technical information on the progress of such an epidemic for consideration by decision makers." The concern here was "to control the spread of the disease," which "may involve measures ranging from direct quarantine to consideration of who would enforce such measures."[19]

Attention to the changing role of the federal government in terrorism preparedness grew in the last years of the Clinton administration and the first months of George W. Bush's presidency. The U.S. Commission on National Security/21st Century (also known as the Hart-Rudman Commission), which started its work in 1998, in 1999 predicted a terrorist attack within the United States. It repeated that warning in its final report, issued shortly after Bush took office. In July, Scott Lillibridge was named special advisor to HHS Secretary Tommy Thompson, and by August 2001 the Bush administration had officially designated FEMA as the agency responsible for "coordinat[ing] federal response efforts in the event of chemical, biological, or nuclear terrorism. In a bioterrorism event, HHS would have special responsibilities, including detecting the disease, investigating the outbreak, and providing stockpile drugs and emergency supplies." At the same time, HHS's Office of Emergency Preparedness expanded the Metropolitan Medical Response Systems and the CDC upgraded its laboratory and epidemiological capacities.[20] Stephen Ostroff of the CDC's National Center for Infectious Disease recalls that "bioterrorism preparedness had only begun receiving funds in 1999. We were still on a steep learning curve in 2001." After 9/11, nearly $1 billion would become available for bioterrorism preparedness. But before then "we only had a couple hundred million dollars — that was all we had. We were questioning whether the pharmaceutical stockpile should be our priority. We were starting from scratch and many of us held the position that it was only so fast that we could have absorbed and used the resources we had effectively."

Bioterrorism preparedness at the federal level was centered in the CDC. Koplan argues that the CDC took the threat of bioterrorism very seriously, and that the organization's "shift in emphasis can be seen in budget allocations" — a shift that began before the terrorist attacks. But the new administration did not support the CDC's efforts. Koplan says that in the first quarter of 2001, when the Health and Human Services budget was announced, reporters "questioned why the NIH received much more money for research on bioterrorism than the CDC received."

According to Koplan, "Tommy Thompson answered, 'We make these kinds of decisions and we think this is proper.'"

The events of 9/11 seemed to end all disagreement over the need to devote more resources to preparing the nation for terrorist attacks of all kinds. Congress at once passed an emergency supplemental appropriation to the CDC's FY 2000 budget that provided $1 billion for terrorism preparedness and $1 billion for smallpox vaccines and drugs. "Then after September 11 we were listened to," Koplan recalls. But despite this apparent unity, divisions over emphasis, priorities, and programs began to emerge almost immediately. In November 2001, the Senate Appropriations Committee's Health Subcommittee heard testimony from Jeffrey Koplan that, according to the *Washington Post,* put "him at odds with his boss [Tommy Thompson] and other Bush administration officials." Koplan testified that the CDC "needs an emergency infusion of nearly $3 billion to prepare for a biological assault," whereas the administration had "requested half that amount for bioterrorism projects such as stockpiling vaccines, upgrading laboratories and expanding surveillance nationwide."[21]

Moreover, it soon became clear that improving bioterrorism preparedness would require much more than budget increases. In December 2001, Larry Gostin and his colleagues published their second draft of the Model State Emergency Health Powers Act, which provided a starting point for discussing the limits of public health surveillance and preparedness. Gene Matthews, then the CDC's legal advisor, remembers that in the late 1990s he "started talking to Larry Gostin about public health law, which had gone unrevised for about fifty years." Daniel Fox, president of the Milbank Memorial Fund, had helped Gostin "think through the role of lawyers both in conversation and in a piece he did in 2000." In 1999, Matthews recalls, he

> had a summer student do a review of laws that could be used to deal with bioterrorism events in the states. We found that most of the laws dated from the 1930s and some were just one sentence long; and in the 1950s, there was no felt need to change these laws because of antibiotics. So alarm bells started ringing and I became concerned. Around this time the Alfred Sloan Foundation asked if they could help, which led to a conference that dealt with homeland security issues. In early 2000, I began to get moving on the public health initiatives and launched the Public Health Law Program in the CDC with academic partners.

From April 2001 to the summer of 2001, he continues, "we laid out a template of how laws needed to be amended. I was concerned that if we had a BT emergency that the federal government could adapt but that the state laws were a patchwork quilt that would need major improvement and no one was looking at that problem. I was concerned because emergencies would devolve to the localities, since they would be making the first detection and the initial remediation."[22]

Matthews believes that the experience of developing the Model Act in the winter of 2001–02 taught the CDC a great deal about public relations; state, local, and federal jurisdictions; and the possibilities and limitations of legal reform. "We were pretty naïve; if we had to do it all over again we would not use the term *model act*. But we were doing something quick and dirty to provide assistance to the states and a template they could use." The CDC was asked, " 'Are you telling the states how to revise their laws?' and we said, 'We are not, but these are the issues you need to look at.' The Model Act was made up out of existing state laws. It was not made up out of thin air. After this it got good traction and the National Conference of State Legislators made a workbook." He adds, "We were surprised at how muted the reaction with regard to civil liberties was. At the time it was very difficult to use the term *quarantine* in public. Larry Gostin brought together the procedural safeguards and protections but we were still surprised that it was not so controversial. After SARS it became crystal clear why you needed quarantine and now it is an acceptable term to use in public."

In March 2002, while various state legislators were considering the Model Act, Jeffrey Koplan resigned as director of the CDC. He explains,

> I never left to be with my family. I said it was time for me to leave. I worked well with Donna Shalala [secretary of HHS, 1993–2001] and wanted to stay on because I'm a passionate CDC advocate and I thought I could get along with anyone. But they [the executive branch] wanted more control and oversight and I didn't think I needed it. Their tone was "You are a renegade and need to be brought into the HHS fold." They got rid of the CDC logo and used the HHS logo. But the staff identity was always with the specific agency. By the summer of 2001 I thought it was reasonable for me to move on. But I wanted to ensure that the budget for the five-year plan was in place. But post-9/11 and anthrax there was no way I wanted to leave and I wanted to make sure that the budget was in place in February 2002. After that, I thought it was in the best interest for the CDC and me to move on because in the absence of full support — and we were not seeing eye to eye — it was not good.

Smallpox Preparedness

In December 2002, President Bush announced the smallpox vaccination program, and in January 2003 he pledged $6 billion for mass vaccination projects and a voluntary smallpox vaccination program for health care workers and public health responders.[23] Joseph Henderson suggests that

> smallpox became a primary focus since it appears as the only disease on CDC's Category A list that is preventable with a vaccine. A vaccine was available to begin immunizations and it could be manufactured in the quantities needed to protect the entire U.S. population. Keep in mind that Category A agents are those that can be easily disseminated or transmitted from person to person; result in high mortality rates and have the potential for major public health impact; might cause public panic and social disruption; and require special action for public health preparedness. In addition to smallpox, Category A agents include plague, botulinum toxin, tularemia, anthrax, and viral hemorrhagic fevers (i.e., Ebola). Since a vaccine was available, then it became evident from the administration that we could take this threat off the table.

Gene Matthews basically supported the view that smallpox had to be taken off the table, declaring that

> the biggest issue was "What is the threat here? Is this a myth or is this real?" I was pretty clear on this. My personal view was that the CDC could not afford to assume that this is not a real threat. We have to go down that path with that assumption. We didn't know if it was a real threat, and I thought the perceived threat was coming from the intelligence community. Mike Osterholm, who had been a state epidemiologist in Minnesota and then an HHS consultant, was part of the team leading the CDC after Koplan left. Prior to September 11, he said that Osama Bin Laden had [weaponized] smallpox. In November 2000, in Washington, D.C., he had talked to the king of Jordan and he said that Osama had smallpox that came out of Russia and that it exists outside of Moscow and the CDC. But even to this day we don't know if that is true. It is these kinds of low-risk, high-consequence issues that drive people in government crazy.

Jeffrey Koplan notes that he

> started in public health in smallpox and had written papers on the disease and on the vaccine. I'm one of only a couple of people in the United States who actually took care of people with smallpox. The issue was, could it be used as a BT agent? WHO's [The World Health Organization's] Dr. D. A. Henderson said it would never be used as a BT agent because it was a poor choice. This was in the 1970s when it was being eradicated. Now there is a different pitch. As CDC director I had briefings and I never heard any convincing evidence that anyone but the U.S. and Russia had it. The ultimate issue was the relative benefit and risk of a vaccination campaign. It made sense to make the vaccine and this started in the 1990s and Tommy Thompson put his weight behind it so that it could be produced in larger quantities. The decision to deploy, quite honestly, made no sense to me. It was not based on knowledge of the disease, how it is controlled in the pres-

ent and how it was controlled in the past. We have an unknown threat of disease and no evidence that anyone else has it. There is a two-week incubation period and we have some allies in its biology and in its control and we have a vaccine.

Koplan adds,

We should have a carefully thought-out plan of how to use the vaccine in a wise and efficient manner. Getting police and firefighters the vaccine made no sense to me. It made as much sense to me as to give the vaccine to your insurance agent. There are real bioterrorism threats to the U.S. population. The more you make these a daily worry for people it can be used for political purposes. If real risks are high, you need to act. But to disproportionately elevate one risk does a disservice to other health risks. Elements in the press, public health, and government used the smallpox scare to have the CDC revert to an old model of infectious diseases. So we did not have to deal with the unpleasant liberal add-ons to the public health agenda such as HIV, obesity, and so on. They said, infectious diseases should be what we're dealing with, not these other services. They wanted to move back the agenda to an earlier era, 1918, 1880, or even earlier, but I think we should do both. These events permit more radical approaches to be taken and the rolling back of where public health is and should be. They want public health narrowly defined and less socially activist.

Joseph Henderson recalls implementing the smallpox vaccine policy as "probably the most complicated thing I have done in my public health career. There was tremendous pressure to prepare the population for a smallpox outbreak, yet it wasn't known initially whether the existing quantities of the vaccine could be stretched to cover the entire U.S. population." He praises Tommy Thompson, who "virtually performed miracles in getting a contract in place to produce new vaccine, but even then it wouldn't be ready for use for many months if not years. In addition to this, there were great concerns about liability, worker compensation, informed consent, assurances that vaccine safety monitoring was adequate and in place, and most importantly lack of confidence in understanding and communicating the real threat or potential of an intentional release of smallpox into our communities. With these issues hanging over our heads, and the emphasis on rapid rollout, short- and long-term program success was difficult to predict." Yet despite "numerous reports that the smallpox vaccination program was a failure," in Henderson's view it resulted in "a number of very important benefits to improving national public health readiness." In May 2003, Congress approved an emergency appropriation of $100 million to support smallpox preparedness, including vaccination of first responders. As a result,

"CDC was able to supplement the state and local bioterrorism prepared-ness and response grants to enhance the focus on smallpox detection, response, treatment, outbreak control, and containment strategies, and vaccine administration and safety monitoring." He argues that these funds had a broader impact because "staff are now trained to administer the vaccine, identify adverse events, set up vaccination clinics to support population-based vaccination, and communicate effectively with the public and health care provider community during a smallpox outbreak. Disease detection, surveillance, and reporting systems have also been improved thanks to the emphasis on smallpox preparedness." Hender-son acknowledges, "We failed to meet the initial vaccination targets," but he declares that "we did not fail to improve national smallpox readi-ness." Ostroff is less certain but also sees benefits in the smallpox cam-paign, noting that it "certainly did not meet the goals that were announced, but the report card is still out. What is interesting is that the military did a phenomenal job and the information we have gathered from that effort has informed our reactions."

George Hardy, a former CDC official who now lobbies for state health officers in Washington, D.C., as executive director of the Association of State and Territorial Health Officers, has a very different take on the smallpox effort:

> It was a disaster! From the day we first heard of it we forgot every lesson we had learned in the swine flu episode [i.e., the national inoculation campaign of 1976] and had to learn these lessons all over again: liability and compen-sation issues were critical. Also, when you make decisions, you have to build in review points — once the first phase is completed, you need to stop, iden-tify the problems, and learn from it. What are your problems? You need to assess. If liability and compensation had been resolved as had been prom-ised, you would probably have had 500,000 inoculated, but because they weren't and there was skepticism over the need for the smallpox program, it failed. There were those who thought that it was a political move by the administration, but others who said, we have to trust what was being said. Most felt it shouldn't be expanded beyond first responders. The reason it was a disaster was that it was cast as a smallpox vaccination program, not a smallpox preparedness program. The states are still supposed to continue with the campaign.[24]

In May 2003, in the midst of the smallpox campaign, TOPOFF 2 took place. The Department of Homeland Security ran this federal exercise, which involved 8,500 government and emergency workers: it simulated the release of pneumonic plague in Chicago and the explosion of a dirty bomb in Seattle. While the Homeland Security secretary told reporters that "the response will be as realistic as possible," independent experts were concerned that "this made-for-television exercise will be more reality TV than reality. Officials will know many details of the attack ahead of time"; and in their opinion that foreknowledge negated the value of the exercise, because "the greatest weapons a terrorist has, after all, are surprise and uncertainty." They compared it to "a final exam where students get a sneak peek at the toughest questions." Frank Hoffman, who had been a top aide to the Hart-Rudman Commission in early 2001, complained that TOPOFF 2 was "too big and too scripted. There's no tolerance for failure. There are no risks being taken. It can't just be all choreographed in advance. You don't test anything."[25] But Richard Jackson points out that however imperfect, these exercises serve a vital purpose: "It is so important to do the drills, the scenarios, the desktops — just going into the field and actually running these episodes in pretend. You have to do it, because that's how you develop — figure out where the gaps are."

STRENGTHS AND WEAKNESSES OF PUBLIC HEALTH RESPONSES TO 9/11

The experiences of September 11, 2001, turned the simulated drills and desktop exercises of the previous few years into tragic reality. In so doing, it revealed the strengths and weaknesses of those earlier planning efforts in ways that could not possibly have been predicted. Ed Thompson argues that 9/11 demonstrated "the capacity of the CDC to deliver the materials from the National Pharmaceutical Stockpile effectively and quickly. We got materials out in seven hours." Stephen Ostroff concurs: "Certain things were started in 1999 that turned out to be right on the mark — the laboratory response network — if we didn't initiate it, the public health system could not have done everything that it did. The other thing was the pharmaceutical stockpile. Before September 11 everyone questioned whether the CDC should organize this. It was actually organized by the NCEH [National Center for Environmental Health], not the ID [National Center for Infectious Disease]. They did an outstanding job and it was critical in the anthrax event."

James Hughes stresses that while federal planning and initiatives are necessary, much of our surveillance system depends on "alert physicians who recognize outbreaks." He points out that "it was an alert physician in south Florida who identified the case of anthrax." Similarly, in Queens, New York, it was an alert local practitioner who identified West

Nile virus; a "doctor at the Navaho reservation in 1993 . . . [who] identified an acute respiratory disease that was found to be caused by a previously unrecognized hantavirus; and clinicians in Hanoi and Hong Kong who noticed SARS." Thompson agrees, noting that "in Florida the diagnosis of anthrax was done well, which showed that private/public cooperation worked well." Certainly, as Hughes points out, planning and infrastructure are necessary, and "communication was improved and that was the most obvious weakness in the system."

It was also apparent that the planning effort had established relatively smooth mechanisms for delivering federal infusions of cash to the states. Ed Thompson recalls that his joining the CDC at the end of February 2002 coincided with "a tremendous infusion of money to the states." The money was allocated with "amazing speed" and, from his point of view, was "spent effectively. As a result of that money, the states are much better prepared. It has increased their emergency response capacity while maintaining other basic services. We got new resources to do emergency response and it did not adversely affect other programs. Initially, we had to take people away from other programs. But then, as we adapted, we were able to deal with other issues such as obesity, child health, etc." Though George Hardy does not foresee that the bioterrorism money will have such profound long-term effects, he does agree that "there was a major concerted effort to do something initially. . . . The HHS got money out the door quickly with very solid guidance, and that's remarkable. Money got out from HHS in a way that no one could have expected." Stephen Ostroff is not sure that the efficient distribution of funds was attributable to pre-9/11 planning but acknowledges that "after September 11 we had a massive infusion of resources . . . and we really did mobilize to accomplish a lot in a year or two." Still, he wonders if it could have been done earlier.

Moreover, public health authorities have increasingly become involved in emergency management. According to Thompson, that relationship "is developing. The departments of emergency management in most states were not initially tied to health but rather to police and fire. These relationships are getting stronger and the states have to see this as being necessary." Accompanying this change have been adjustments in the law. Not until the trauma of 9/11 did public health authorities seriously reconsider the legal structures upon which their authority to act was based. Historically, it has rested in state and local statutes, which often evolved very haphazardly and addressed only local problems and concerns; the result was a patchwork quilt of state, local, and federal laws and authority. September 11 "has empowered states to look at the laws and the issues," says Gene Matthews:

> They realized that if there was an emergency we need to have the tools — including laws — to deal with that emergency. About forty states have used the Model Law to change the laws. Should you have a one-size-fits-all statute because we have a federal system? But when the bioterrorism infrastructure money — $2 billion — went out to the states, we were able to tack on a provision that the states need to look at their laws and we were able to deliver the toolkit to the states to do so. For example, Georgia had a one-sentence law and now they have a fairly comprehensive statute.

James Hughes notes that the infusion of funds improved not just the public health infrastructure but the physical plant of the CDC itself,

> after years of neglect. A new building opened up here with new lab space right before the anthrax attack. But many other components on the laboratory side are not really adequate. We have new buildings scheduled for completion next spring [in 2005]. We have a bio 3 level lab. The only disease to be eradicated was smallpox but we have spent a lot of time and money on it! There is more work to do than people to do it. The increases in resources are tied to crises of the moment. We got supplements for West Nile and SARS. And we are looking for money to strengthen local and state activities. Antimicrobial drug resistance is a major, major issue.

One new federal program that has a great deal of promise is "BioSense," which Stephen Ostroff describes as "an information-gathering endeavor looking for data streams and sources of better information of possible BT events." He adds, "We are developing a syndromic surveillance system on a national scale. This has caused a small problem with local health departments because resources that used to go to them are now going to the CDC." According to Hughes, another benefit of BioSense is that it "began to try to bridge the gulf between clinical care and public health," thereby addressing a long-standing "need to get the two cultures together." After all, so many of today's threats transcend the traditional boundaries between population and personal health, even extending to the boundaries between humans and animal diseases — and "issues of zoonotic disease" underscore the need for veterinarians to become involved with the public health community. Thus the events of September 11 and the threat of bioterrorism have forced a reevaluation of the boundaries of public health itself.

One sign that we have learned a great deal from our experience is the relatively efficient and effective responses of the public health community to more recent threats of infectious disease. "Have things improved since anthrax?" asks Ostroff. "Things are absolutely better. Just think about our reaction to SARS, monkeypox, and influenza — we were out in front on those things. Now it is like night and day." Hughes agrees that "we are better prepared to detect infectious disease threats, and better prepared than before SARS. We have a close relationship with WHO and global health is an important part of our mission. We wouldn't have had as effective a response to the SARS outbreak five or six years ago." Even Scott Lillibridge, a persistent critic of the CDC, calls the agency's reaction to SARS "top-notch" (and a "sharp contrast to their response to BT").

As Joseph Henderson explains,

> Thanks to the lessons learned from the 2001 anthrax response, CDC was much better positioned to support the global SARS outbreak. In January 2003, CDC opened their new Emergency Operation Center. This facility was built to support cross-agency management of CDC responses. This in addition to the permanent placement of trained EOC staff and the development of policies and procedures to support agency-wide response set the stage for CDC's response to SARS. As a result, CDC was better positioned to play the lead role in the U.S. response; communications with the Department of Health and Human Services, Homeland Security, state and local public health agencies, and the World Health Organization were better coordinated; and communicating with the public became an essential component of CDC's response. It should also be noted that improved capacities were apparent at the state and local levels of the public health system during the SARS response. States such as Washington and California were much better able to ramp up their surveillance systems to detect SARS cases and report them to local health agencies as a result of post-9/11 capacity building.

Thompson, Lillibridge, and Henderson all agree with Ostroff's declaration: "We are more secure in that the public health system is much better prepared to recognize and respond to potential threats. I can't think of any area where we are less secure other than the general problem that it is very difficult to prepare for every eventuality." "In every way we are more secure," Thompson argues. "In almost no way are we less secure. The stockpile, emergency response and communication, the emergency operations protocol, the Health Alert Network system, and communications and state labs have been renovated." Perhaps Richard Jackson's summary of the lessons learned from 9/11 is the most poignant: "This is frightening stuff. I remember going home just agitated sometimes, listening to this. What happens if somebody takes a lecture bottle, which is a small compressed canister of hydrogen sulfide or something else, and sets it off in the Times Square third-level shuttle? What kind of Q & As — what kind of protocols do we need to have? What kind of training do we have to have people have in advance?" He finds that the theoretical issues that dominated the TOPOFF exercises as well as Dark Winter and other desktop scenarios are now all too real, and all needed to be considered: "What are my risks of going through the radiologic and chemical scenarios? The biological scenarios were being taken care of by the infectious disease group. We spent a lot of time thinking the unthinkable, and a lot of this is in place. It's not sitting on a website, but it's ready for when it occurs."

The federal response to 9/11 revealed real and important strengths; but as the crisis recedes from the nation's collective memory and as federal budget deficits vitiate the promise of substantial improvements in the population health infrastructure, federal officials are raising concerns about the country's ability to defend itself against future bioterrorist attacks. Richard Jackson, speaking about six months after 9/11, expressed optimism about the "big opportunity" to address deficiencies in "the infrastructure of public health": "The pipeline of young leaders, how we support and train them, how we pay for communications systems, how we have a common data system for reporting of illnesses, and how we have a common data system for reporting of environmental hazards — it is a complete Tower of Babel, and here's a real opportunity to fix this." He believed that such repairs are essential, because "perhaps 99.99 percent of the emergencies that occur in the future will not be terrorist-related. The degree to which we can take this warning and fix the infrastructure so that they can deal with the immense majority of these episodes that are not terrorism — if you can deal with the train spill, if you can deal with the more routine, if you will, catastrophes, well, you're in a much better position for then dealing with the terrorist catastrophe when it comes."

Amy Smithson, director of the Chemical and Biological Weapons Nonproliferation and Response Project at the Henry L. Stimson Center, criticized the federal government's priorities immediately following the attacks. While the revised budget devoted $9.7 billion to terrorism preparedness in FY 2001, only $100 million of that sum was devoted to public health infrastructure and surveillance. In November 2001, she said that "the federal government has got it bass-ackwards to date. . . . They do not seem to comprehend that lives are saved in a disaster by locals."[26] Gene Matthews amplifies her point: "Where we are now is that we're beginning to forget why Congress provided all the money. For example, Vermont is concerned that 20 percent of the bioterrorism money is now going to be going to the cities. We are earmarking money for metropolitan targets. At first, we were told that we needed to build up the state public health system and the states were saying that if we start whittling it down we can't do what we need to do." Joseph Henderson, speaking almost three years after the attack, worries that

> critical public health programs such as childhood immunization and chronic diseases continue to see ups and downs relative to year-to-year funding — bioterrorism funding could easily follow that same trajectory. State and local public health agencies are seeing record-low funding levels to support public health and few states in the country are appropriating funds to support emergency public health preparedness. The federal government is truly the only large funding source for this activity, and should these funds be realigned to address new priorities the public health infrastructure supported by these dollars will rapidly crumble. The threat continues to exist, even if real evidence is lacking to prove it. The Soviet Union produced tons of weapons-grade anthrax, much of which is still not accounted for. Dissemination of this material does not require sophisticated delivery systems. The threat of nuclear terrorism continues to grow as technologies are shared and the producers of fissionable material increase. However, the U.S. and the world are much more likely to experience a natural event such as influenza or SARS. Regardless of the threat, we must get prepared now if we are to truly survive a potential catastrophe.

George Hardy points to "the effect of the worsening budget situation on public health. . . . In the last few months the federal government initiated the CRI [Cities Readiness Initiative]," which, Stephen Ostroff explains, is aimed at making "sure major cities around the country are able to distribute antibiotics in a period of forty-eight hours." Hardy acknowledges that

> the initiative itself is good, but the funding is inadequate. The idea behind CRI is that, for example, aerosolized anthrax is not that difficult to create, so they have given money to twenty-one cities to plan and drill to get antibiotics to everyone. . . . You can argue whether the number of cities is good or bad, but what the federal government did was take $1 billion from every state from their programs. Thus every state is taking a 22 percent reduction from smallpox campaigns, the SRP [Stockpile Reliability Program] stockpile. So, local government is now maintaining that they are not getting resources for maintaining the stockpile, and BT in general, and CRI. States got a bundle of money but it is too diffused. Local government feels the states are not giving enough. For 2005 it has been proposed to take $105 million from the states for BioSense, a new federal initiative, but without any new funding. So you have a 22 percent reduction next year, a $105 million mandated program, and CRI that already exists, plus new cities that are being added on to CRI. Now they say we need to strengthen local safety labs, improve mental health programs. SAMHSA [Substance Abuse and Mental Health Services] is telling locals to go to the state for resources

and the states are being given more responsibility by the feds, but there are no new resources.

According to Hardy, the federal budget crisis led to a schism between Washington politicians and the recipients of federal money. First, budget hawks sought to delay payments of money that had been promised to the states. Then, when money allocated to different state agencies was spent, the lag between its use by the states and the auditing and reporting process allowed federal officials and politicians in Washington to argue that the money had in fact not been spent and therefore the following year's appropriation for the states should be curtailed. He notes,

> There are a couple of issues: initially the money went out on a needs basis. The feds said we have established bank accounts in each state. But with CRI and anthrax . . . there has been a constant change in focus. There are huge frustrations in the states, the federal government justifies shifting dollars to CRI by saying that states are just not spending the money. But there are two things wrong with this: the states spend the money and can draw down from the feds, but they need to bill the feds and get payments later — as much as a year later. They have to file financial status reports where states say what was spent and what is owed. In fact states spent or obligated 92 percent of money in the first year. The feds have the data, but the feds don't use it because it is not "audited." Congress has been told that the states are not spending and then they are forced to reappropriate the money, so this justifies not appropriating new money. The secretary of HHS and Bush say that the states are not spending the money, and this is coming from the secretary's office. His staff has briefed him, we know, but this is a mantra that the secretary uses to justify not going back to Congress for more money.

In a formal statement made public in November 2004, the Association of State and Territorial Health Officials concluded that collectively the states had spent over 90 percent of CDC and HRSA funds but that there was "often a delay of several months between the time a state expends funds and then recovers those costs through the federal 'draw down' process. As a result of this delay, 'draw down' analyses frequently reflect far lower figures than the actual situation within the states."[27]

Hardy argues that

> the problem is just that there is no new money — the president won't ask Congress and the Congress won't appropriate it, so it is mutually reinforcing. Everything is a shell game right now. Today, we announce initiatives and next week we announce other initiatives using old money. The constant refrain for the last twenty years has been "Don't trust government" and people, surprise, don't. The biggest long-term problem is that you can't get smart young people to go into government. We have so devalued

government service — every major politician campaigns against government — that fewer and fewer young people consider careers in government. This is frightening.

He adds, "What's happened subsequently because of the shrinking federal budget is more disturbing. Because of the ongoing deficit, bioterrorism, and so on, the discretionary funds are fewer and fewer. There is no political will to sustain spending and with every new need identified, the pressure is increasingly being shifted to the states." Richard Jackson worries "that we are being much too aggressive about buying things we can put on a shelf, and nowhere near aggressive enough about improving the minds, training, and skills of the people that will have to manage these episodes. It's nowhere near as impressive. People look the same at the end of these trainings as they do at the beginning of the trainings, but you live or die on the quality of your people when you're responding to these episodes."

Gene Matthews identifies the ongoing problems that declines in trust and funding create for bioterrorism preparedness. "We are better prepared but the question is 'What is the perceived threat?' . . . There is a good deal of questioning and lower tendency to believe the government and that is problematic from a public health point of view. In another crisis a public health official needs to look at the camera and say 'We need to take this action'; and when the government doesn't have credibility, it is much harder to do that." He fears that the growing distrust of government will spread to a distrust of public health officials, which could have a disastrous effect during future crises: "What happened in Toronto with the quarantining of tens of thousands of citizens [because of SARS] was amazing and the question is, would we have the level of cooperation that they did? If you don't have some level of trust, it's going to make it more difficult the next time we have a crisis."

Maintaining confidence in health agencies becomes all the more important because Matthews and other federal officials consider an attack a question not of if but of when. Further, they foresee even more ominous methods of attack, which will test public trust in government and its agencies even more severely. Jackson describes a couple of possible scenarios:

> I fear that another one is coming, whether chemical or radiologic. I actually fear that more than bioterrorism. I think there's been too much emphasis on bio, and not enough — the chemical scenarios, and we spent three months after the World Trade Center event — by "we" I mean my center — thinking

the unthinkable. What happens if someone steals cesium and flies an airplane into the Empire State Building? What happens? — it's not that hard to get hold of cesium or strontium or medical radiologic waste. What happens if one of the eighty missing suitcase nuclear devices from the Soviet Union arrives in a container ship in the Potomac?

The looming issue relevant to addressing bioterrorism is the public's trust in the statements and actions of its political leaders as well as public health officials. "I'm very concerned about the budget crises," Matthews explains. "The public was very forgiving after 9/11, anthrax, etc. and very tolerant of its leaders. But the thing the public expects now of their governments is that they have their acts together. I say to the business community, 'If there is another emergency, the business community cannot afford for the government to fail.' We are facing triple budget deficits at the local, state, and federal levels, so we are primed to fail because resources are being cut back and we don't have the resources to properly prepare."

Jeffrey Koplan is a bit more specific in assessing the problems for public health infrastructure resulting from an increasing focus on bioterrorism: "We are a public health agency, not a part of the military. We had a culture where it was easy to have interchanges among scientists and we realized the need to reach out to the community. The bioterrorism concerns were real but were at odds with the ways of public health's doing things. By its very nature bioterrorism has close ties to law enforcement and the military. Public health does not have close ties to these institutions but rather seeks ties to community groups." He points out that for at least the past two generations, mutual trust between public health officials and communities has been nurtured and has grown. But the concentration on bioterrorism emphasizes the police powers of the public health community. Such activities as surveillance and disease reporting and tracking worry community groups concerned with civil liberties and intrusions on privacy. Conversely, those focused on bioterrorism criticize the isolation of, for example, public health surveillance activities from homeland defense as putting the country at risk. Koplan explains, "When we focus on one it is quite jarring to the other." But he sees the trend over the past four years as "an increasing emphasis of the military basis of public health. People [in the U.S. Public Health Service] are wearing uniforms more frequently and increasingly thinking of themselves as part of the uniformed services. This is different from the CDC and the NIH. This might seem like a superficial issue but causes morale issues and affects recruitment of new individuals and retention of people who have other options. It has an effect on the quality of the workforce." Koplan believes that funding cuts for programs not related to bioterrorism, such as those addressing chronic diseases and obesity, are connected to "the militarization of public health."

Hardy concurs with Koplan's analysis that "the cultural differences between public health workers and other first responders are great." For "the best example" of this split, he turns to the case of anthrax in Florida, "a singular event investigated by law enforcement and public health people." On the one hand, "the public health culture is premised on the idea that you get as much information out as possible, as quickly as possible and share it with the world. That way others can help you identify outbreaks and incidents." On the other hand, "law enforcement goes in and gets information and clamps the lid on it. They have different cultures and the different cultures clash. One is premised on openness and the other is based on secrecy and preserving information in confidence." For Hardy, "one of the concerns is that public health clearly has to work with law enforcement and does have to be privy to secret information. But the concern expressed by a number of agencies is that many of the people that public health works with are marginalized persons — undocumented workers, people with AIDS, and others who distrust law enforcement because of the possible repercussions of deportation, or issues of privacy."

While the possible breakdown in public trust threatens public health services, Hardy argues that there are also real benefits to the new attention to the influence of the military on public health bureaucracies. "The biggest problem in public health is how leaders respond in times of crisis. I have helped develop a national preparedness leadership initiative with the Kennedy School and the School of Public Health at Harvard . . . for forty officials in public health, emergency preparedness, and senior staffers in Congress. We have not had leaders bold enough to take the right moves at the right time. This is the weakest link in the chain."

PUBLIC HEALTH AND THE DEPARTMENT OF HOMELAND SECURITY

In November 2002, Congress passed a bill creating the Department of Homeland Security, a cabinet-level agency that incorporated twenty-two existing federal agencies, including FEMA, the Immigration and Naturalization Service, the Secret Service, the Customs Service, the Transportation Security Administration, and the Border Patrol. Tom Ridge, former governor of Pennsylvania, became the department's first secretary in January 2003.

The ideological disagreements about the best focus for public health play out in the relationship between public health officials and the Department of Homeland Security. While Ed Thompson argues that this relationship "is developing," George Hardy sees "good and bad things in the establishment of the DHS — one of the really good things is that Homeland Security is really eager to learn about public health — what it does and how to include it in their thinking. Hence public health is much more integrated into the state response apparatus than ever before." Stephen Ostroff's "impression is that they have had a variable relationship. There have been bumps in the road. In some areas it has worked very well, but in other areas there have been challenges. I think it is mostly due to the rapidity of the growth and differences over who should be responsible for things like the stockpile. The BioWatch program is funded by Homeland Security and it has the lead, but the CDC and HHS are the implementers. That is a problem. We are all on a steep learning curve." Initially, the various agencies struggled over where public health activities would sit. Joseph Henderson recalls that the "CDC did not want [the administration] to strip disease out of the CDC and it was able to maintain its independence and the Department of Homeland Security kept its hands off both the CDC and the NIH. This was, in part, because both research and the practical response was with state and local authorities." Ironically, he sees "the strongest resistance" to the CDC's relative independence in the Department of Health and Human Services. "It's been a difficult journey for us because the department does not understand what the public health system really does. . . . The department does not understand the battlefield."

Henderson believes that eventually the personal trust between Tom Ridge at Homeland Security and Julie Gerberding at the CDC overcame institutional tensions; in his view, the two agencies "work well together because Ridge and Gerberding have a tremendous relationship." Even so, as Hardy points out, "there are problems: the BioWatch program (started at EPA) has caused problems in some places." In New York City Marci Layton, the city's assistant commissioner for communicable disease, "agreed to monitor and put the program into effect, but some planners simply said 'We'll send specimens to the public health labs,' and there was no planning as to who would pay for the laboratory services and who would coordinate activities." Hardy observes that despite the goodwill of New York's Department of Health personnel, federal officials gave "no thought as to who would pay and take responsibility," leaving the city with a tremendous burden.

IS OUR BIOTERRORISM PREPAREDNESS BEING EVALUATED?

When George Hardy was asked about ongoing assessments of the recent changes in bioterrorism preparedness, he answered: "This question gets to the biggest problems: a couple of years ago the hospitals said that we need $11 billion to improve and develop services. They knew what their deficits were, and what they needed from their own perspective. But public health cannot answer that question, because we haven't agreed on what we are planning for. There are too many arbitrary indicators and there are no agreed-upon indices of success or accountability. If we don't know where we are going, we can't say what we need and what it will cost." What is most critical, he says, is that "we need to have a definition of what we are preparing for. What is the risk? Is it anthrax? An explosion? In NYC the mayor says that it is unfair for NYC to get a much smaller per capita budget for terrorism preparedness than North Dakota. But North Dakota says that a crop duster filled with anthrax that flies over a stadium filled with 80,000 people is just as dangerous as anything that might happen in NYC. What about nuclear power plants or agroterrorism?"

The Trust for America's Health study of bioterrorism preparedness concluded that the "policy is ill-defined and inconsistent" and that the "planning still lacks strategic direction, well-defined priorities and appropriate levels of resources to match the needs." It also found that "shifting federal priorities and programs are distracting from fixing fundamentals."[28] Ed Thompson is more sanguine: "We are in the process of doing [good evaluation] right now. We are piloting means to measure and means of assuring accountability. We established critical benchmarks on the grant money that was distributed and we are asking states to tell us if they have achieved those benchmarks and if not, when they will. We are in the process of developing a measurement-based evidence system to see if we have been effective." Joseph Henderson concurs:

> We are trying to establish with the states performance indicators and to be able to define the gaps so that we can go back to Congress to help us establish performance indicators to help find out if a highly suspicious event needs to be responded to and if labs capacity is adequate, for example. We are now looking at systems so that they can be appraised or criticized. We are trying to find the problems and to mobilize to address them. Surveillance

is meaningless in a vacuum. We need to know what is the real problem, what is the appropriate response, and then what is needed to return to a normal state.

One problem is that there are few benchmarks by which to measure progress. The lack of standardization among the various states makes it hard to measure whether essential public health functions such as surveillance, reporting, or even access to public health authorities have improved since 9/11. Because virtually all public health practice is local and no federal requirements for disease reporting or other essential functions are in place, it is difficult to evaluate to what degree we may now be better prepared for a bioterrorist attack. Our interviews make clear that communication between agencies such as fire, police, and public health has generally improved, but the fact remains that such improvements are uneven. The GAO reported in 2004 that in a number of specific areas, states' preparedness has improved; for example, states had put in place executive directors of local bioterrorist preparedness and response programs, and 90 percent of the population was covered by the Health Alert Network. But the GAO also found that few states met two of the CDC's "critical benchmarks": developing a "statewide response plan for incidents of bioterrorism and other public health threats and emergencies and provisions for exercising the plan" or developing a "regional response plan across state borders for incidents of bioterrorism and other public health threats and emergencies."[29]

CONCLUSION

What Lessons Have We Learned?

What lessons are to be drawn from this historical account? September 11 presented the public health community and those involved with population health more generally an immense opportunity to revitalize and rethink the nation's health agenda. Politicians, administrators, and the general public came to appreciate the vital role that public health agencies could play in a national emergency and in the fight against terrorism; public health administrators and advocates hoped that they could perhaps recapture the importance and promise that they believed their field had once possessed. Some observers called for revamping the nation's health insurance system to cover more of the population as a means of improving the surveillance of disease; some called for expanding the scope of traditional public health activities to lower the growing barriers between prevention and care; some called for extending the social service system and integrating it with the health care and public health systems; and some called for upgrading the public health infrastructure as necessary in the fight against terrorism. Others cautioned that simply increasing budgets and financial resources might do little to address the long-term problems affecting public and population health programs in the various states. While those in general government — elected officials and members of their staff — and public health agencies agreed on many points, the former had little interest in addressing decades of problems in public health departments by increasing the funding for their activities generally.

Much of the success of the public health response to 9/11 in New York City had less to do with formal emergency planning or conscious preparation than with the presence of an existing infrastructure of health services, laboratories, and personnel. Though many officials outside the city praised New York's ability to take action during the crisis, and some personalized its success by attributing it to the political leadership, in fact the work was done by bureaucracies that nothing and no one could have mobilized had they not already been there.

A second major lesson of New York City's experience is that we need to develop a more expansive understanding of mental health services and integrate our current, individualized system more broadly into our public health infrastructure. In fact, on July 1, 2002, the city's Department of Health merged with the Department of Mental Health to become the Department of Health and Mental Hygiene. It becomes clear, once we acknowledge the broad impact of terrorism on the mental health of society, that all people affected — from schoolchildren in the immediate area of the attack on the World Trade Center to their parents, neighborhood residents, and anyone directly touched by the tragedy — deserve comprehensive mental health care, regardless of their income or private insurance coverage. This recognition has the potential to lead to a huge transformation in how we conceive of our society's responsibilities to those in need. Whether this challenge to our broader assumptions about who is "worthy" and who is "unworthy" of care will gain strength or will fade remains to be seen. An ancillary point is that we need a much better understanding of how best to respond to a population's social and economic needs in a crisis. The public health and social welfare communities initially responded to the trauma of 9/11 by abandoning practices of the past decades — indeed, the past century — that had often inhibited access to a variety of services. Immediately following the attack, a more open system of social services was instituted. However, this early promise of broader rights to health and social welfare services, irrespective of income, was soon lost.

A third message that comes through loud and clear is that failure to communicate honestly about uncertainty is a big mistake. The issuance of pronouncements that obviously are not supported by everyday observations will in the end backfire, as the public officials making such claims are certain to lose the public's trust and goodwill and ultimately their authority. Human beings will persist in believing that air that smells and makes us cough is not good for us, no matter what experts or political leaders say about the lack of danger as indicated by scientific investigations.

Finally, the attacks of September 11, 2001, were on the nation, not just New York City, the Pentagon, or Pennsylvania. When national threats are present, clear lines of federal and other authority need to be established. A cacophony of voices does not serve the public well or use resources efficiently. Local authority need not be usurped, but decisive leaders who control resources and make decisions with good personal and situational intelligence are required in times of crisis. In the anthrax event, where there was clear leadership (e.g., that of Mayor Rudy Giuliani), the system worked reasonably well. When many jurisdictions operated within their narrow preserves, communicating poorly and competing for primacy, the system fell apart.

In examining the public health community's response in the various states, we conclude that even as "emergency response" is in the process of being defined, the purview of public health must continue to expand, helping professionals in the field to understand the breadth of social and medical activities that determine a population's health and well-being. For much of the past century, public health officials, politicians, and administrators of city agencies in general clung to very traditional notions of what constituted dangers to the public's health, which they addressed in discrete functions: sanitation, emergency care, scientific data collection, and surveillance. But in recent decades this narrow definition of public responsibility began to give way, a process accelerated considerably by the events of the past five years, which have forced government officials — indeed, all of us — to rethink what health is, which agencies are responsible for a population's health, and what the public's role is in defining an environment as healthful or unhealthful.

In response, government officials at the state and local levels paid attention to a broad array of social service, public health, and health care needs, each with its claim on scarce state and federal resources. Public health officials focused on the possibility of improving the traditional infrastructure of their agencies, including lab capacity, surveillance systems, lines of intra- and interagency communication, and processes for protecting the borders. Certainly, the mobilization around public health needs led to the allocation of significant resources and to what many of those to whom we spoke called "progress." After September 11, 2001, officials and legislators in state government were buffeted by geopolitical events and federal decisions that dramatically altered the basic assumptions under which they had long operated. Rural county officials, often isolated and laboring far from state as well as federal seats of power, could hardly be expected to be fully prepared for their new responsibilities for developing plans to defend against a bioterrorist or chemical attack. At the state level, legislators and officials responsible for population health and well-being had to attend to an extensive array of needs at a time when resources were scarce.

In the early months after the attacks and the anthrax episodes, those concerned about public health in America believed that the new resources supplied by the federal government could be used to address long-standing infrastructure weaknesses as well as to meet the new antiterrorism mandates. State officials were accustomed to some "cause of the day" receiving massive funding for a year or two and then being forgotten, but they believed that this time it would be different, that the profound shock of 9/11 would lead to equally profound changes. Many state officials anticipated that the federal government would finally fund public and population health programs at a level that would protect citizens not only from narrowly defined bioterrorist threats but also from SARS and other infectious diseases. Some even hoped for general improvements in health care and the availability of health insurance. There was no intrinsic contradiction between the traditional goals of public health departments — such as investigating and monitoring illnesses, studying them in the laboratory, and providing well-baby services and health care for the uninsured — and the new goal of participating as full members in an emergency response team. Officials in general government and those in public health agencies agreed on many of the same goals — but state legislators and their staffs had to create balanced budgets that devoted about 80 percent of their expenditures to entitlement programs (such as Medicaid), whereas those in public health agencies sought to maintain programs more traditionally associated with preventive services.

Media coverage, our interviews, and reports both published and unpublished make clear that in the years since 9/11, much has been done to provide more resources, begin needed legal reform, improve surveillance, and enhance communications. The focus of the Centers for Disease Control and Prevention (CDC) and Health Resources and Services Administration programs has expanded beyond smallpox and preparations for war against Iraq, while their grant programs demonstrate that the federal government remains committed to addressing all forms of terrorism: the amounts awarded in fiscal years 2003, 2004, and 2005 match those in 2002. The strengthening of the public health infrastructure (together with employment growth as the country recovers from a recession) has resulted in a modest improvement in access to health care, general childhood inoculation programs, well-baby services, and mental health care. It has also aided the coordination of emergency response within and between agencies; in some communities, laboratory capacity has improved. According to the CDC, federal initiatives, grants, and programs have resulted in a number of significant improvements in public health preparedness within individual states.

Through its own grants, the CDC has fostered the development of surveillance systems, management information systems, interagency cooperative agreements, and twenty-four-hour-a-day public health emergency response systems; it has also identified physicians who, in an emergency, will serve as consultants in diagnosing and treating infectious diseases. Among its accomplishments are stronger relationships between law enforcement officers and health providers, enhanced epidemiological and laboratory capacity, better training for possible bioterrorist events, improved and more secure communication systems, and successful inoculation of a group of health professionals who are now capable of responding to a smallpox outbreak. Joseph Henderson, a CDC senior management official, notes, "In 2005, CDC will be awarding $862,777,000 to support state and local public health response efforts. Since these funds are intended to enhance detection and surveillance capabilities, improve laboratory diagnostic capacities, improve the delivery and quality of workforce training, improve outbreak control and containment strategies, and enable improved communication, it goes without saying that the basic public health infrastructure benefits from these investments."[1]

Certain bioterrorism-specific reforms will undoubtedly remain, but the early optimism fueled by new federal interest and funding has waned as state legislators, governors, and public health officials all have come up against state and federal budget crises and a falloff of federal attention. Legislators in most states have had to make hard choices in allocating their reduced moneys for education, social welfare, direct health services, and population health more generally. Real funding increases are needed to build up the public health infrastructure sufficiently for these departments to shoulder the new burden of countering terrorism and bioterrorism. Many public health officials were bitterly disappointed that the apparent federal commitment to these upgrades vanished as memories of September 11 began to fade. The nation's public and population health infrastructure unquestionably has suffered as a consequence of the Bush administration's repeated insistence to the nation that Iraq was the focal point of the real war on terrorism — and therefore of our budget priorities. And many perceived a schism between those who favored a narrow focus on smallpox and those who argued for building up defenses against bioterrorism in general and strengthening long-term population health. As Dennis Perrotta of Texas points out, "The small-pox vaccination effort in many jurisdictions was seen as a distraction from basic preparedness and public health activities. The growth of this area seemed incongruent with the significant losses of population health programs as states and state health departments faced fiscal conditions of unparalleled instability."[2]

State officials vary in their confidence that their states will be able to ride out the budget problems currently hobbling their public and popu-lation health programs. Further, some are concerned that in the long run, emergency preparedness will be impaired by a weakened public health system. Michael Caldwell, commissioner of the Dutchess County, New York, Department of Health and former president of the National Association of County and City Health Officials, says, "Most public health professionals do not look at the bioterrorism money to solve all our social ills, but to expand our 'dual-use,' which means surveillance and response functions of communicable diseases."[3] But as the Govern-ment Accountability Office recently confirmed, others worry that the massive shift of resources into traditional emergency response areas such as fire departments and law enforcement will detract from the pressing needs of the medical and public health sectors and impair their ability to detect and respond to bioterrorism. A Council of State and Territorial Epidemiologists report recommended that "dual use of terrorism and emergency preparedness epidemiology resources should be substantially expanded to realign functional roles and build overall capacity of state health departments to prepare for and respond to terrorism, infectious disease outbreaks, and other public health threats and emergencies."[4]

Many in general government feared that a narrow focus on health as an adjunct to national defense could undermine health agencies' broader mission to provide a variety of services not necessarily tied to bioterror-ism and emergency preparedness. The economic recessions that in some states had begun before 9/11 strained state budgets and forced spending reductions for many state functions, including health. As time passed, the need to respond to the events of late 2001 seemed less urgent and popu-lation health preparedness became just one of a number of different budget priorities that legislators had to consider in tough fiscal times. The budgetary problems were magnified by the federal mandate in late 2002 to institute a major smallpox inoculation campaign.

The attempt to codify and reformulate state public health laws with the draft Model State Emergency Health Powers Act, together with what some criticized as the poor federal handling of the anthrax episode and smallpox inoculation campaign, served to stimulate a broad discussion of the new obligations and responsibilities of health authorities. Some worried that an emphasis on surveillance techniques and disease reporting, though long a part of public health management, might undermine public trust in the system as a whole if seen as an infringement on personal liberties. In the aftermath of September 11, the clash of conflicting values — setting the rights of individuals against the perceived need for greater bioterrorism preparedness — has heightened the sense of disorder for officials already dealing with the swift and radical transformation of their jobs.

The federal government, through the CDC, has accomplished a great deal in its efforts to improve emergency response and bioterrorism preparedness. Notably, in addition to aiding individual states and cities, it has expanded the National Laboratory Response Network, increased the Strategic National Stockpile of pharmaceuticals and medical supplies and ensured their delivery to any place in the United States within twelve hours, and developed new technologies for more effective systems of surveillance and data sharing. But, as Joseph Henderson puts it, "The key concern today is to assure that federal, state, and government leaders and elected officials don't sacrifice the ground gained since September 11 due to new priorities and shifting political interests. Significant resources are in place to support broad-based public health including public health readiness. One cannot exist without the other. A solid public health system strives to reduce/eliminate illness, injury, and death every day but especially when a catastrophic event occurs such as bioterrorism or SARS."

Maintaining the public health infrastructure is probably the single most important means of preparing the nation for the myriad unpredictable crises arising from naturally occurring epidemics as well as from terrorist attacks. Without a strong permanent infrastructure, the best emergency planning will be inadequate. The financial difficulties of the various states, combined with the federal government's shift in focus from bioterrorism and terrorism in general to smallpox and the war in Iraq in particular, have lessened the chance of achieving what had seemed likely immediately after 9/11: enhancement of the system of services that are essential to improve national bioterrorism preparedness and to address the overall health needs of the American people.

NOTES

PREFACE

1. Texas State Senator Leticia Van de Putte, telephone interview by Gerald Markowitz and David Rosner, September 12, 2005.

2. Jane Bullock, quoted in S. B. Glasser and J. White, "Storm Exposed Disarray at the Top," *Washington Post*, September 4, 2005, A1.

3. Timothy J. Roemer, quoted in ibid.

INTRODUCTION

1. Richard Jackson, interview by David Rosner and Gerald Markowitz, May 17, 2002. All subsequent quotations from Jackson are from this interview.

2. Jeffrey Koplan, telephone interview by Gerald Markowitz and David Rosner, June 30, 2004.

3. T. G. Thompson, "Bioterrorism: We Are Prepared, But We Can Do Better," *Vital Speeches of the Day* 68, no. 1 (2001): 6–8.

4. Gene Matthews, telephone interview by Gerald Markowitz and David Rosner, July 6, 2004.

5. For these working definitions of the scope of public and population health, we have depended on D. M. Fox, "Populations and the Law: The Changing Scope of Health Policy," *Journal of Law, Medicine & Ethics* 31 (2003): 607–14.

6. James Hughes, telephone interview by Gerald Markowitz and David Rosner, October 12, 2004.

1. SEPTEMBER 11 AND SHIFTING PRIORITIES

1. D. M. Fox, foreword to *Public Health Administration: Principles for Population-Based Management*, edited by L. F. Novick and G. P. Mays (Gaithersburg, Md.: Aspen, 2001), p. xix.

2. J. L. Bruno, "New York's Emergency Response Plan Tested by Terrorism," *Spectrum: The Journal of State Government*, Fall 2001, pp. 7–8.

3. In addition to devoting resources to the existing public health infrastructure, New York supported the development of the Health Insurance Plan of New York (HIP) and Blue Cross; the expansion of health department clinics, public hospitals, and public housing; the nation's largest public university system; and what was, until the 1980s, often considered a generous welfare system. See, for the post–World War II years, J. Freeman, *Working-Class New York: Life and Labor since World War II* (New York: New Press, 2000).

4. Richard Gottfried, interview by Valerie Kiesig, July 10, 2002; subsequent quotations from Gottfried are from this interview. The original states in the compact were California, Wyoming, Hawaii, and Arkansas.

5. Kelly McKinney, interview by Sheena Morrison, June 12, 2002. All subsequent quotations from McKinney are from this interview.

6. Doris Varlese, interview by Valerie Kiesig, July 22, 2002. All subsequent quotations from Varlese are from this interview.

7. Susan Waltman, interview by Valerie Kiesig, July 22, 2002.

8. Richard Jackson, interview by Gerald Markowitz and David Rosner, May 17, 2002.

9. Susan Blank, interview by Nancy VanDevanter, January 3, 2002. All subsequent quotations from Blank are from this interview.

10. Lucindy Williams, interview by Sheena Morrison, May 28, 2002. All subsequent quotations from Lucindy Williams are from this interview.

11. Isaac Weisfuse, interview by David Rosner, January 14, 2002. All subsequent quotations from Weisfuse are from this interview.

12. Benjamin Mojica, interview by David Rosner, January 16, 2002. Subsequent quotations from Mojica are from this interview.

13. New York City Department of Health, Office of Public Affairs, "In Response to the World Trade Center Disaster," press release, September 16, 2001 (available at www.nyc.gov/html/doh/html/press_archive01/pr79–916.shtml; accessed December 6, 2005); Thomas R. Frieden, Commissioner, NYC Department of Health, and Joel A. Miele, Commissioner, NYC Department of Environmental Protection, testimony before the U.S. Senate Committee on Environment and Public Works, Subcommittee on Clean Air, Wetlands, and Climate Change, 107th Cong., 2nd sess., February 11, 2002 (available at www.nyenvirolaw.org/PDF/DOH-DEP-2-11-02-TestimonyForSenateHearing.pdf; accessed December 6, 2005). Because it was displaced from its headquarters, the department oversaw the re-creation of a system to collect and protect vital records, including birth and death certificates.

14. Andrew Goodman, interview by Nancy VanDevanter, January 2, 2002; Goodman, post-interview comments, November 7, 2002.

15. McKinney interview.

16. The entire infrastructure of public health training was threatened as well. In the 1980s, many schools of public health had seemed on the brink of closure, including those at Harvard and UCLA; since then, these institutions have recovered and the number of schools of public health has indeed increased, not fallen. In New York, it was not until the late 1990s that Columbia's Mailman School of Public Health gained a relatively stable source of income, after the donation of a gift created an endowment.

17. J. Steinhauer and J. Dwyer, "FBI Did Not Test Letters to NBC or Immediately Notify City Hall," *New York Times,* October 13, 2001, A1.

18. Samuel Sebiyam, interview by Valerie Kiesig, June 6, 2002.

19. S. Kershaw, "Defense Dept. Aids a Busy City Health Agency with Tests," *New York Times,* October 22, 2001, B8.

20. L. Garrett, "Overwhelming Challenge," *Newsday,* October 21, 2001, A6.

21. E. Goode, "Anthrax Offers Lessons in How to Handle Bad News," *New York Times,* October 23, 2001, F1.

22. Ibid.; S. G. Stolberg, "On Many Fronts, Experts Plan for the Unthinkable: Biowarfare," *New York Times,* October 23, 2001, F4.

23. Steven Rubin, interview by Sheena Morrison, June 12, 2002. All subsequent quotations from Rubin are from this interview.

24. David Klasfeld, interview by David Rosner and Gerald Markowitz, June 6, 2002. All subsequent quotations from Klasfeld are from this interview.

25. A. Gendar, "Stuyvesant HS Planning Stringent Tests for Asbestos," *Daily News,* September 28, 2001, p. 6.

26. A. Gendar, "Traces of Asbestos Further Setback for HS: Findings Could Delay Stuyvesant Re-opening," *Daily News,* September 29, 2001, p. 9.

27. Molly Rosner and student friends, conversations with David Rosner, October 3–12, 2001.

28. J. Williams and E. Hays, "Stuyvesant Re-opens, But Students Jittery," *Daily News,* October 10, 2001, p. 27.

29. M. Rosner conversations.

30. A. Gendar, "Stuyvesant under Scrutiny: Levy Sending Experts to Find Cause of Ailments," *Daily News,* October 10, 2001, p. 35; David Rosner, conversations with parents, October 2001–February 2002.

31. Jacqueline Moline, quoted in Gendar, "Stuyvesant under Scrutiny."

32. K. Roth, "School Officials Still Unsure What's Causing Illness," Associated Press State and Local Wire, October 18, 2001.

33. J. Williams, "Post-9/11 Ills Found at HS; Many Stuyvesant Staffers Suffered," *Daily News,* May 11, 2002, p. 7.

34. D. Rosner conversations.

35. Barbara Aaron, interview by Rochelle Frounfelker, August 15, 2002. All subsequent quotations from Aaron are from this interview.

36. D. Cardwell, "Workers and Residents Are Safe, Officials Say," *New York Times,* November 2, 2001, B10.

37. Department of Health and Christine Todd Whitman, quoted in A. Katz, "Toxic Haste: New York's Media Rush to Judgment on New York's Air," *American Prospect,* February 25, 2002, p. 13.

38. Cardwell, "Workers and Residents Are Safe, Officials Say," B10.

39. Ibid. The same article attributes to Robert Adams, director of environmental health and safety services for New York's Department of Design and Construction, the claim that "although workers at the [WTC] site were still required to wear respirators and other protective gear, the data suggest that even an unprotected worker would not experience long-term health risks from the levels of poisons that had been detected."

40. Jerrold Nadler, interview by Valerie Kiesig, July 12, 2002. Unless otherwise specified, all subsequent quotations from Nadler are from this interview.

41. J. Gonzalez, "A Toxic Nightmare at Disaster Site," *Daily News,* October 26, 2001, p. 2.

42. Marc Ameruso, quoted in Cardwell, "Workers and Residents Are Safe, Officials Say," B10.

43. Stanley Michels, quoted in ibid.

44. J. Williams, "Public Distrusts Gov't Air Tests," *Daily News,* November 21, 2001, p. 23.

45. J. Gonzalez, "Hostile Environment Near WTC," *Daily News,* December 20, 2001, p. 32.

46. S. Q. Stranahan, "The Health of Ground Zero," *Milwaukee Journal,* January 24, 2002, p. 11A.

47. Katz, "Toxic Haste," p. 13.

48. S. Davidsdottir, "Smokescreen: Ground Zero Has Officially Been Cleared . . . ," *Guardian* (London), June 5, 2002, p. 8.

49. Ekaterina Malievskaia, post-interview comment, November 13, 2002.

50. A. Schneider, "NY Officials Underestimate Danger," *St. Louis Post-Dispatch,* January 13, 2002, p. 1.

51. K. Johnson, "Air Testing After Sept. 11 Attack Is Both Perplexing and Reassuring," *New York Times,* May 15, 2002, A1.

52. K. Johnson, "With Uncertainty Filling the Air, 9/11 Health Risks Are Debated," *New York Times,* February 8, 2002, A1.

53. "Congressman 'Outraged' by EPA's Response to September 11," *Occupational Hazards* 64 (April 2002): 22.

54. Nadler interview; see also Jerrold Nadler, "White Paper — Lower Manhattan Air Quality" (mimeograph), April 12, 2002.

55. Johnson, "With Uncertainty Filling the Air, 9/11 Health Risks Are Debated," A1.

56. A. Gendar and G. Gittrich, "Feds to Foot $11.7M Bill for School WTC Clean-up," *Daily News,* June 4, 2002, p. 10.

57. Joel Kupferman, quoted in D. Fagin, "Safety Took a Backseat," *Newsday,* November 4, 2001, A42.

58. Ekaterina Malievskaia, interview by Rochelle Frounfelker, August 5, 2002. All subsequent quotations from Malievskaia are from this interview.

59. Newspapers throughout the country were beginning to take notice; see Stranahan, "The Health of Ground Zero."

60. Steven Markowitz, quoted in Johnson, "Air Testing After Sept. 11 Attack Is Both Perplexing and Reassuring," A1.

61. Malievskaia interview.

62. EPA Office of Inspector General, "EPA's Response to the World Trade Center Collapse: Challenges, Successes, and Areas for Improvement," Report Number 2003-P-00012, August 21, 2003, www.epa.gov/oig/reports/2003/WTC _report_20030821.pdf (accessed June 14, 2005), pp. 1, 111, 21.

63. Sierra Club, "Air Pollution (and Deception) at Ground Zero," August 18, 2004, www.sierraclub.org/groundzero (accessed June 14, 2005).

64. Igal Jellinek, interview by Rochelle Frounfelker, July 18, 2002. Unless otherwise specified, all subsequent quotations from Jellinek are from this interview.

65. I. Jellinek, "Perspectives from the Private Sector on Emergency Preparedness for Seniors and Persons with Disabilities in New York City," statement before the U.S. Senate Special Committee on Aging, 107th Cong., 2nd sess., February 11, 2002 (available at http://cscs-ny.org/ussenatetestimony.html; accessed December 6, 2005).

66. Ibid.

67. Jack Krauskopf, interview by Rochelle Frounfelker, June 7, 2002. Unless otherwise specified, subsequent quotations from Krauskopf are from this interview.

68. September 11th Fund, "The September 11th Fund: The First Six Months" (New York, 2002), available at www.september11fund.org/six_month _report.pdf (accessed December 6, 2005).

69. S. Strom, "Red Cross to Open Its Books on Aid After Sept. 11," *New York Times*, June 5, 2002, B7.

70. Eliot Spitzer, quoted in R. Rabin, "The War on Terror," *Newsday*, November 8, 2001, A36.

71. L. H. Sun, "Red Cross to Give All Funds to Victims," *Washington Post*, November 15, 2001, A1. American Red Cross President Bernadine Healy resigned at about this time. By 2002, approximately $2 billion had been collected, almost half of which was raised by the Red Cross and almost one-quarter by the September 11th Fund. Other organizations that collected more than $50 million include the New York Firefighters 9–11 Disaster Relief Fund, the Twin Towers Fund, the Salvation Army, the Uniformed Firefighters Association's Widows' and Children's Fund, New York State World Trade Center Relief Fund, New York Times 9/11 Neediest Fund, and the Robin Hood Relief Fund; the last is the only one of these funds specifically targeted at low-income victims of the disaster. See S. Strom, "Families Fret as Charities Hold a Billion Dollars in 9/11 Aid," *New York Times*, June 23, 2002, A29.

72. By October 7, the estimated amount of donations had increased to more than $1 billion. By October 30, estimates grew to $1.2 billion. And as of June 21, 2002, it was over $2 billion. See S. Saul, "As Record Donations Pour In, Non-Profits Struggle to Disperse It," *Newsday*, October 7, 2001, A5; "Charity and Red Tape" (editorial), *New York Times*, October 30, 2001, A16; S. Strom, "Families Fret as Charities Hold a Billion Dollars in 9/11 Aid," *New York Times*, June 23, 2002, A29.

73. K. Shatzkin, "Red Cross Declines to Take Part in Charities' Victim Data Base," *Baltimore Sun*, September 28, 2001, p. 6A.

74. "Collaborative Charity" (editorial), *New York Times*, October 15, 2001, A18; see also S. Saul, "Red Cross to Share Grantee Lists," *Newsday*, October 25, 2001, A37.

75. S. Saul, "Umbrella Group Hopes to Cut Red Tape," *Newsday,* December 15, 2001, A19.

76. Jack Krauskopf, post-interview comment, November 14, 2002.

77. C. E. Steuerle, "Managing Charitable Giving in the Wake of Disaster," *Charting Civil Society,* no. 12 (May 2002): 2.

78. Mimi Abramovitz laid out at length the argument for broad distribution of charity in her interview by Rochelle Frounfelker, June 3, 2002. Unless otherwise specified, all subsequent quotations from Abramovitz are from this interview.

79. E. Auster, "What to Do with All That Money?" *Cleveland Plain Dealer,* October 7, 2001, A1.

80. E. Wyatt, "At Ground Zero, a New Divide," *New York Times,* June 5, 2002, B1.

81. City of New York, "Executive Budget: Fiscal Year 2003, Budget Summary" (New York: Office of Management and Budget, 2002); United Way of New York City, *Beyond Ground Zero: Challenges and Implications for Human Services in New York City Post September 11* (New York: United Way of New York, 2002), p. 40 (available at http://unitedwaynyc.org/?id=69#; accessed December 6, 2005).

82. "A Hunger Emergency in New York" (editorial), *New York Times,* November 26, 2001, A16.

83. Fiscal Policy Institute, "World Trade Center Job Impacts Take a Heavy Toll on Low-Wage Workers," prepared for the New York City Central Labor Council and the Consortium for Labor Education (New York: Fiscal Policy Institute, 2001), table 3; see also charts, pp. 8, 9 (available at www.fiscalpolicy.org/Nov5WTCreport.PDF; accessed December 6, 2005).

84. Abramovitz interview; see also M. Abramovitz, *In Jeopardy: The Impact of Welfare Reform on Non-Profit Human Service Agencies in New York City,* Task Force on Welfare Reform, New York City Chapter, National Association of Social Workers (New York: United Way of New York City, 2002), p. 10.

85. Ibid., p. 11. Some estimated that 50,000 New Yorkers would be thrown off welfare and onto the job market in the three months following the WTC disaster; see R. Schachter, "Another Fallout from the Disaster: Social Problems Will Become Even Less Visible," Executive Director's Reports, New York City Chapter of the National Association of Social Workers, October 2001 (available at www.naswnyc.org/ex11.html; accessed December 6, 2005).

86. Independent Sector, *A Survey of Charitable Giving after September 11, 2001* (Washington, D.C.: Independent Sector, 2001), p. 1.

87. Abramovitz interview.

88. Jellinek interview; post-interview comment, December 2, 2002.

89. Independent Sector, *A Survey of Charitable Giving after September 11, 2001,* p. 2.

90. Douglas Gould and Company, survey; cited in United Way of New York City, *Beyond Ground Zero,* p. 40.

91. Mother Martha Overall, quoted in J. Martinez, "Grim Fight to Feed the Poor: Food Lines Longer as City Reels from 9/11," *Daily News,* January 6, 2002, p. 1 (suburban ed.).

92. "A Hunger Emergency in New York," A16.

93. C. Lee, "The Other Disaster," *Village Voice,* October 16, 2001, p. 26.

94. A. Townsend, "The Crisis for Non-Profits," *Crain's New York Business,* October 1, 2001, p. 9.

95. Steuerle, "Managing Charitable Giving in the Wake of Disaster"; see also Independent Sector, *A Survey of Charitable Giving after September 11, 2001.*

96. New York City Department of Mental Health, Office of Public Affairs, "Following the World Trade Center Disaster, the New York City Department of Mental Health Provides Services for Those in Need," press release, September 18, 2001.

97. K.C., personal communication with David Rosner, September 23, 2001.

98. New York City Department of Mental Health, Office of Public Affairs, "Commissioner Neal L. Cohen, M.D., Submits Testimony to U.S. Senate Committee on Psychological Trauma and Terrorism," press release, September 28, 2001.

99. P. O'Brien, "Statement on Hospitals' Response to Mental Health Needs in the Aftermath of the World Trade Center Disaster," delivered at a public hearing of the New York City Council's Subcommittee on Mental Health, Mental Retardation, Alcoholism and Drug Services, November 8, 2001 (available at www.gnyha.org/testimony/2001/pt20011108.html; accessed December 7, 2005).

100. New York City Department of Mental Health, "Following the World Trade Center Disaster."

101. M. Gormley, "Free Counseling Offered to New Yorkers Coping with September 11," Associated Press State and Local Wire, November 7, 2001.

102. S. Galea, J. Ahern, H. Resnick, D. Kilpatrick, M. Bucavalas, J. Gold, and D. Vlahov, "Psychological Sequelae of the September 11 Terrorist Attacks in New York City," *New England Journal of Medicine* 346 (2002): 982–87.

103. J. Purnick, "Metro Matters: Portraits of Trauma," *New York Times,* May 20, 2002, B1; see also N. R. Kleinfield, "In Nightmares and Anger, Children Pay Hidden Cost of 9/11," *New York Times,* May 14, 2002, B1.

104. A. Goodnough, "Arts Groups Helping Schools Deal with Disaster," *New York Times,* November 14, 2001, D12.

105. O'Brien, "Statement on Hospitals' Response to Mental Health Needs."

106. Ezra Susser, interview by Rochelle Frounfelker, August 5, 2002. All subsequent quotations from Susser are from this interview.

107. Rubin interview.

108. L. Williams interview.

109. K. A. Ballard and J. Cataldo, "Statement of the New York State Nurses Association before the [New York State] Assembly Committees on Health and Codes on Public Health Emergency Planning and Response and the Model State Emergency Health Powers Act," March 14, 2002.

110. W. Lopez, "Testimony before the New York State Assembly Committees on Health and Codes on Public Health Emergency Planning and Response and the Model State Emergency Health Powers Act," March 14, 2002.

111. Gail Nayowith, interviewed by Rochelle Frounfelker, June 21, 2002. All subsequent quotations from Nayowith are from this interview.

112. The September 11th Fund, "Grants by Category as of 12/1/04," in "About the Fund," www.september11fund.org/aboutus.php (accessed December 31, 2005).

2. EMERGENCY PREPAREDNESS AND THE STATES

1. J. Schwartz, "Efforts to Calm the Nation's Fears Spin Out of Control," *New York Times,* October 28, 2001, p. 4; L. Copeland, "Local Public Health Officials Seek Help," *USA Today,* October 23, 2001, A3; N. Kristof, "This Is Not a Test," *New York Times,* December 28, 2001, A19; C. Burress, "State Can't Handle Bioterrorist Attack," *San Francisco Chronicle,* November 7, 2001, A11; T. Abate, "Scared into Action," *San Francisco Chronicle,* October 8, 2001, E1; C. Connolly, "Public Health System Is on War Footing," *Washington Post,* October 27, 2001, A1.

2. G. Evans, B. Clements, and B. Shadel, "We Can't Fight Bioterrorism on the Cheap," *St. Louis Post-Dispatch,* November 28, 2001, B7.

3. S. Satel, "Public Health? Forget It; Cosmic Issues Beckon," *Wall Street Journal,* December 13, 2001, A6.

4. Tommy Thompson, quoted in C. Terhune, "Public Health Officials Say More Funding, Information Needed to Fight Bioterrorism," *Wall Street Journal,* October 23, 2001, B8.

5. Satel, "Public Health? Forget It," A6.

6. Mohammed Akhtar, quoted in S. E. Christian, "Anthrax Scare; Health System's Weakness Exposed," *Chicago Tribune,* November 18, 2001, p. 1.

7. Robert Stroube to Kate Frank, e-mail, "Emergency Preparedness, Bioterrorism, and the States," October 30, 2003. See also N. B. King, "Security, Disease, Commerce: Ideologies of Post-Colonial Global Health," *Social Studies of Science* 32 (2002): 763–89; E. W. Etheridge, *Sentinel for Health: A History of the Centers for Disease Control* (Berkeley: University of California Press, 1992); E. Fee, "Public Health and the State: The United States," in *The History of Public Health and the Modern State,* edited by D. Porter (Amsterdam: Rodopi, 1994), 224–75; A. D. Langmuir and J. M. Andrews, "Biological Warfare Defense 2: The Epidemic Intelligence Service of the Communicable Disease Center," *American Journal of Public Health* 42 (1952): 235–38.

8. See N. B. King, "The Influence of Anxiety: September 11, Bioterrorism, and American Public Health," *Journal of the History of Medicine* 58 (2003): 433–41; B. Rosenkrantz, *Public Health and the State* (Cambridge, Mass.: Harvard University Press, 1972); D. Rosner, ed., *Hives of Sickness: Public Health and Epidemics in New York City* (New Brunswick, N.J.: Rutgers University Press, 1995); C. Sellers, "September 11 and the History of Hazard," *Journal of the History of Medicine* 58 (2003): 449–58; and N. Tomes, *The Gospel of Germs: Men, Women, and the Microbe in American Life* (Cambridge, Mass.: Harvard University Press, 1998), and "Reflections on September 11: A Symposium," *Journal of the History of Medicine* 58 (2003): 428–32.

9. Stroube to Frank, e-mail.

10. This brief overview of public health draws on J. M. Colmers and D. M. Fox, "The Politics of Emergency Health Powers and the Isolation of Public Health," *American Journal of Public Health* 93 (2003): 392–99; M. J. Coye, "Our Own Worst Enemy: Obstacles to Improving the Health of the Public," in *Leadership in Public Health,* edited by M. J. Coye, W. H. Foege, and W. L. Roper (New York: Milbank Memorial Fund, 1994), available at www.milbank.org/

reports/mrlead.html#fore (accessed December 7, 2005); L. O. Gostin, "Public Health Law in an Age of Terrorism: Rethinking Individual Rights and Common Goods," *Health Affairs* 21 (2002): 79; and Rosner, ed., *Hives of Sickness,* especially E. Blackmar, "Accountability for Public Health: Regulating the Housing Market in 19th-Century New York City," 42–64; G. A. Condran, "Changing Patterns of Epidemic Disease in New York City," 27–41; and D. M. Fox, "The Politics of Public Health in New York City," 197–210.

11. Anne Harnish, interview by Gerald Markowitz and David Rosner, April 1, 2003. All subsequent quotations from Harnish are from this interview.

12. Ronald Cates, interview by Gerald Markowitz and David Rosner, April 4, 2003. All subsequent quotations from Cates are from this interview.

13. Harriette Chandler and Tim Daly, interview by Gerald Markowitz and David Rosner, April 15, 2003. All subsequent quotations from Chandler and Daly are from this interview.

14. Angela Coron, interview by Gerald Markowitz and David Rosner, April 2, 2003. All subsequent quotations from Coron are from this interview.

15. Dennis Perrotta, interview by Gerald Markowitz and David Rosner, April 10, 2003. All subsequent quotations from Perrotta are from this interview.

16. Catherine Eden and David Engelthaler, interview by Gerald Markowitz and David Rosner, March 21, 2003. Unless otherwise specified, all subsequent quotations from Eden and Engelthaler are from this interview.

17. Mary Kramer, interview by Gerald Markowitz and David Rosner, April 11, 2003. All subsequent quotations from Kramer are from this interview.

18. Rice Leach, interview by Gerald Markowitz and David Rosner, March 19, 2003. Unless otherwise specified, all subsequent quotations from Leach are from this interview.

19. Rice Leach, quoted in C. Wolfe, "Kentucky Plans Possible Bioterrorism Response," *Cincinnati Enquirer,* June 10, 2002.

20. Anthony Moulton, interview by Gerald Markowitz and David Rosner, April 2, 2003.

21. T. V. Inglesby, R. Grossman, and T. O'Toole, "A Plague on Your City: Observations from TOPOFF," *Clinical Infectious Diseases* 32 (2001): 436.

22. Richard Raymond, response to draft report, ca. December 2003.

23. ANSER Institute for Homeland Security, "Dark Winter," July 2003, www.homelandsecurity.org/darkwinter/index.cfm (accessed July 29, 2003).

24. Norma Gyle, interview by Gerald Markowitz and David Rosner, April 8, 2003. All subsequent quotes from Gyle are from this interview.

25. Philip Lee, quoted in S. Russell, "Public Health Care under a Microscope: Bioterror Attacks Bring New Focus to Neglected Facilities," *San Francisco Chronicle,* December 2, 2001, A6.

26. T. Seibert, "Bioterror to Be Top Priority for Grant; State Makes Plans for $16.3 Million," *Denver Post,* April 2, 2002, B3. On the condition of labs in California and Colorado, see J. Graham, "Money Woes Plague Nation's Health Labs," *Chicago Tribune,* November 23, 2001, p. 23.

27. Gyle interview.

28. Warren Wollschlager, quoted in G. Condon, "Hospitals Team Up against Terrorism," *Hartford Courant,* November 15, 2002.

29. Georges Benjamin, quoted in S. H. Thompson, "Knowledge May Serve as Public Health Antidote to Bioterrorism Worries," *Tampa Tribune,* October 21, 2001, p. 9.

30. J. Nesmith, "Health Systems' Bioterror Readiness Up," *Atlanta Journal and Constitution,* November 13, 2002, p. 13A.

31. Benjamin, quoted in Thompson, "Knowledge May Serve as Public Health Antidote," p. 9.

32. See Christian, "Anthrax Scare; Health System's Weakness Exposed"; A. Hajat, C. K. Brown, and M. R. Fraser, "Local Public Health Agency Infrastructure: A Chartbook," October 2001, http://archive.naccho.org/documents/chartbook _frontmatter1–2.pdf (accessed November 5, 2003).

33. Georges Benjamin, interview by Gerald Markowitz and David Rosner, March 12, 2003.

34. Centers for Disease Control and Prevention, Media Relations, Office of Communication, "Fact Sheet: Public Health Infrastructure," May 14, 2002, www.cdc.gov/od/oc/media/pressrel/fs020514.htm (accessed December 7, 2005).

35. Centers for Disease Control and Prevention, "Public Health's Infrastructure: A Status Report Prepared for the Appropriations Committee" (2001), pp. iii, 3. See also K. Eban, "Waiting for Bioterror: Is Our Public Health System Ready?" *The Nation,* December 9, 2002, pp. 11–18.

36. R. Kampeas, "States Adjust to Governing with Threat of Bioterror," *North County Times,* June 19, 2002; available at www.NCTimes.net (accessed December 7, 2005).

37. Graham, "Money Woes Plague Nation's Health Labs," p. 23.

38. Department of Health and Human Services, "HHS Announces $1.1 Billion in Funding to States for Bioterrorism Preparedness," press release, January 31, 2002; available at www.hhs.gov/news/press/2002pres/20020131b.html (accessed December 7, 2005).

39. Centers for Disease Control and Prevention, "CDC and HRSA Bioterrorism and Response Grants, Illinois Homeland Security," 2002, www.100.state .il.us/security/ittf/terrorismreport14.htm (accessed November 23, 2003). See also State of Maryland, Governor's Press Office, "Governor Glendening Announces Maryland Awarded More than $19 Million for Anti-Terrorism Efforts," June 6, 2002, available at www.dhmh.state.md.us/publ-rel/html/pro60602.htm (accessed December 7, 2005); S. G. Stolberg, "U.S. Will Give States $1 Billion to Improve Bioterrorism Defense," *New York Times,* January 25, 2002, A11.

40. M. Guiden, "Public Health Officials Prep for Bioterror with New Hires," *Stateline.org,* September 6, 2002, available at www.stateline.org (accessed December 7, 2005).

41. A. Staiti, A. Katz, and J. F. Hoadley, "Has Bioterrorism Preparedness Improved Public Health?" Center for Studying Health System Change, Issue Brief no. 65 (July 2003), at www.hschange.org/CONTENT/588/ (accessed December 7, 2005).

42. Stroube to Frank, e-mail.

43. Guiden, "Public Health Officials Prep for Bioterror with New Hires."

44. Ibid.

45. Melvin Neufeld, interview by Gerald Markowitz and David Rosner, March 11, 2003. All subsequent quotations from Neufeld are from this interview.

46. M. L. Boulton, J. Abellera, J. Lemmings, and L. Robinson, "Brief Report: Terrorism and Emergency Preparedness in State and Territorial Public Health Department — United States, 2004," *Morbidity Mortality Weekly Reports* 54 (2005): 459–60.

47. Richard Falkenrath, James M. Hughes, and David Satcher, quoted in S. J. J. Freedberg and M. W. Serafini, "Be Afraid, Be Moderately Afraid," *National Journal* 31 (1999): 812–13.

48. Mary Selecky, quoted in Guiden, "Public Health Officials Prep for Bioterror with New Hires."

49. Christian, "Anthrax Scare; Health System's Weakness Exposed," p. 1.

50. "Bioterrorism Preparedness and Response: A Connecticut Approach" (n.d.); courtesy of Norma Gyle.

51. Ohio Department of Health, "State Bioterrorism Preparedness Capacity: Key Accomplishments" (March 2003).

52. Harnish interview.

53. Ohio Department of Health, "State Bioterrorism Preparedness Capacity."

54. Virginia Department of Health, "State Bioterrorism Preparedness Capacity: Key Accomplishments" (March 2003).

55. "Funds Boost Public Health Preparedness," *Emergency Management Update,* ca. September 6, 2002, p. 6.

56. Lisa Kaplowitz, interview by Gerald Markowitz and David Rosner, March 11, 2003. Unless otherwise specified, all subsequent quotations from Kaplowitz are from this interview.

57. "Health Department Reports Progress on Emergency Preparedness," *Virginia Town and City* 37 (2002): 1–2.

58. Sheila Peterson, interview by Gerald Markowitz and David Rosner, April 2, 2003. Unless otherwise specified, all subsequent quotations from Peterson are from this interview.

59. Arvy Smith and Brenda Vossler, interview by Gerald Markowitz and David Rosner, April 9, 2003. All subsequent quotations from Smith and Vossler are from this interview.

60. Kentucky Department of Health, "State Bioterrorism Preparedness Capacity: Key Accomplishments" (March 2003).

61. Wolfe, "Kentucky Plans Possible Bioterrorism Response."

62. Seibert, "Bioterror to Be Top Priority for Grant," B3.

63. Neufeld interview; J. Thomas Schedler, interview by Gerald Markowitz and David Rosner, April 17, 2003 (all subsequent quotations from Schedler are from this interview).

64. George DiFerdinando, Jr., interview by Gerald Markowitz and David Rosner, April 4, 2003. Unless otherwise specified, all subsequent quotations from DiFerdinando are from this interview.

65. E. A. Bresnitz and G. DiFerdinando, "Lessons from the Anthrax Attacks of 2001: The New Jersey Experience," *Clinics in Occupational and Environmental Medicine* 2 (2003): 227, 240.

66. Ibid., p. 243.

67. Jack Colley, interview by Gerald Markowitz and David Rosner, April 9, 2003. All subsequent quotations from Colley are from this interview.

68. "Terrorism: Are We Prepared?" *County Magazine* [Texas Association of Counties], January/February 2002, www.county.org/resources/library/county _mag/county/141/5.html (accessed December 8, 2005).

69. Perrotta interview; see also C. Mabin, "Lawmakers Updated on State's Bioterrorism Plans," Associated Press State and Local Wire, January 29, 2002; "Texas Department of Health Maintaining Readiness in Case of Bioterrorist Act, Associated Press State and Local Wire, September 28, 2001.

70. W. Welsh, "Homeland Security Gets Shortchanged," *Washington Technology,* March 10, 2003, www.washingtontechnology.com/news/17_23/statelocal/ 20257–1.html [accessed September 8, 2003]).

71. "Terrorism: Are We Prepared?"

72. S. G. Stolberg, "The President's Budget Proposal: Buckets for Bioterrorism, But Less for Catalogue of Ills," *New York Times,* February 5, 2002, A20.

73. Georges Benjamin and Leslie M. Beitsch, quoted in Stolberg, "U.S. Will Give States $1 Billion to Improve Bioterrorism Defense," A11.

74. Lee Greenfield, interview by Gerald Markowitz and David Rosner, April 16, 2003. All subsequent quotations from Greenfield are from this interview.

75. J. M. Colmers, S. D. Pattison, and S. Peterson, "State Health Expenditures Before and After September 11th," ms in authors' possession.

76. Outside reviewer, anonymous comments on draft, October 31, 2003.

77. Minnesota Council of Non-Profits, "Impact of the Final FY 2004–05 Budget," MN Budget Project, August 14, 2003, www.mncn.org/doc/fy200405 .pdf (accessed December 8, 2005).

78. Mary Selecky to Kate Frank, e-mail, "Milbank Report Review," November 3, 2003.

79. "State Budget Shortfall Map," *NOW with Bill Moyers,* January 10, 2003, www.pbs.org/now/politics/budgetmap.html#ar (accessed December 8, 2005); N. Johnson and B. Zahradnik, "State Budget Deficits Projected for Fiscal Year 2005," Center on Budget and Policy Priorities, revised February 6, 2004, www.cbpp.org/10–22–03sfp2.htm (accessed January 8, 2006).

80. California Budget Project, "The 2003–04 Budget Gap: Where Are We after the May Revision and the Budget Conference Committee?" June 30, 2003, www.cbp.org/2003/030516WhereAreWeMayRevise.pdf (accessed December 8, 2005).

81. Charlene Rydell, interview by Gerald Markowitz and David Rosner, April 17, 2003. All subsequent quotations from Rydell are from this interview.

82. Trust for America's Health, *Ready or Not? Protecting the Public's Health in the Age of Bioterrorism 2004,* December 14, 2004, http://healthyamericans .org/reports/bioterror04 (accessed December 12, 2005).

83. Colmers, Pattison, and Peterson, "State Health Expenditures Before and After September 11th."

84. M. W. Walsh and M. Freudenheim, "Huge Rise Looms for Health Care in City's Budget," *New York Tmes,* December 26, 2005, A1.

85. Robert B. Eadie, interview by Gerald Markowitz and David Rosner, March 21, 2003. All subsequent quotations from Eadie are from this interview.

86. Russell, "Public Health Care under a Microscope," A6.

87. Catherine Eden, comments on draft, ca. December 2003.

88. Catherine Eden, quoted in P. Davenport, "State Releases Plan to Vaccinate Some Health Workers for Smallpox," Associated Press State and Local Wire, December 10, 2002; Lisa Kaplowitz, quoted in A. Hostetler, "Virginia Submits Smallpox Plan," *Richmond Times-Dispatch,* December 10, 2002, A1.

89. Schedler interview; DiFerdinando interview.

90. D. G. McNeil, "National Programs to Vaccinate for Smallpox Come to a Halt," *New York Times,* June 19, 2003, A13.

91. Dennis Perrotta, quoted in M. A. Roser, "Smallpox: Is the U.S. Vaccination Program a Shot in the Arm for Anti-Terrorism or a Shot in the Dark by the White House?" *Austin American-Statesman,* January 19, 2003, E1.

92. Interviews with Leach, Eden and Engelthaler, and Kaplowitz.

93. Gene Matthews, telephone interview by Gerald Markowitz and David Rosner, July 6, 2004.

94. Joseph Henderson, telephone interview by David Rosner and Gerald Markowitz, June 29, 2004.

95. Ed Thompson, telephone interview by David Rosner and Gerald Markowitz, July 7, 2004.

96. Greenfield interview; Harnish interview.

97. Lisa Kaplowitz, quoted in A. Manning, "Two Soldiers Develop Bad Reactions to Smallpox Shot," *USA Today,* February 5, 2003.

98. Leach interview; "Public Health Commissioner Gets Smallpox Vaccine," Associated Press State and Local Wire, January 30, 2003.

99. "Federal Agency Approves Smallpox Vaccinations," Associated Press State and Local Wire, December 28, 2002.

100. State of Wisconsin, "Smallpox Planning and Vaccination Strategies," Region V State Health Officials Meeting, October 30, 2002; courtesy of John Chapin.

101. Benjamin interview.

102. Joseph Hunt to Kate Frank, e-mail, October 28, 2003.

103. J. Nick Baird to Andrew Gyory, e-mail, October 28, 2003.

104. J. Chapin, "Presentation to Public Health Assembly Committee, Dr. Frank Urban, chair," October 22, 2001.

105. K. Murphy, "Preparedness Found Lacking in Rural Areas," *Milwaukee Journal Sentinel,* October 22, 2001.

106. Chapin, "Presentation to Public Health Assembly Committee."

107. John Chapin, interview by Gerald Markowitz and David Rosner, March 3, 2003.

108. J. Chapin, "How Can Public Health Be Funded for Bioterrorism and Still Be Public Health?"; memorandum to Public Health Partners Developing Your Budget on Bioterrorism (an ad hoc group of Wisconsin public health officials), November 8, 2001.

109. Chapin interview.

110. Chapin, "How Can Public Health Be Funded for Bioterrorism and Still Be Public Health?"

111. J. Chapin, "Funding Prerequisites for Public Health," memorandum, October 18, 2001; courtesy of John Chapin.

112. J. Chapin, "Reflections on Public Health and the War on Terrorism," typescript, June 15, 2002.

113. Chapin interview.

114. Chapin, "Funding Prerequisites for Public Health."

115. "Terrorism Experts Speak of Readiness," *Beloit (Wisc.) Daily News,* October 23, 2001.

116. Chapin, "Reflections on Public Health and the War on Terrorism."

117. State of Wisconsin, "Motions and Actions Taken by the Board, Wisconsin State Laboratory of Hygiene Board Meeting," University of Wisconsin Center for Health Sciences, March 26, 2002.

118. Chapin, "Reflections on Public Health and the War on Terrorism."

119. Chapin interview.

120. Chapin, "How Can Public Health Be Funded for Bioterrorism and Still Be Public Health?"

121. Chapin interview.

122. Ibid.

123. J. Chapin, "Wisconsin Concerns," typescript, ca. October 2002.

124. Chapin interview.

125. Colmers and Fox, "The Politics of Emergency Health Powers and the Isolation of Public Health"; Gostin, "Public Health Law in an Age of Terrorism"; L. O. Gostin, J. W. Sapsin, S. P. Teret, and S. Burris, "The Model State Emergency Health Powers Act: Planning for and Response to Bioterrorism and Naturally Occurring Infectious Diseases," *Journal of the American Medical Association* 288 (2002): 622–29.

126. Anthony Moulton to Kate Frank, e-mail, "Review Comments on Rosner-Markowitz Draft," October 20, 2003.

127. NACCHO, "Turning Point," www.naccho.org/topics/infrastructure/TurningPoint.ctm (accessed June 2005).

128. "Law Makers Not Keen on 'Model' Public Health Law," quoted in R. Bayer and J. Colgrove, "Rights and Dangers: Bioterrorism and the Ideologies of Public Health," in *In the Wake of Terror: Medicine and Morality in a Time of Crisis,* edited by J. D. Moreno (Cambridge, Mass.: MIT Press, 2003), p. 64; see also Guiden, "Public Health Officials Prep for Bioterror with New Hires."

129. Daniel Fox, "Interview with Ron Bayer," March 7, 2002; quoted in Bayer and Colgrove, "Rights and Dangers," p. 64.

130. Bayer and Colgrove, "Rights and Dangers," p. 65.

131. Moulton to Frank, e-mail; Bayer and Colgrove, "Rights and Dangers," pp. 64–65; and J. G. Hodge, Jr., and L. O. Gostin, "Protecting the Public's Health in an Era of Bioterrorism: The Model State Emergency Health Powers Act," in Moreno, ed., *In the Wake of Terror,* pp. 17–32.

132. S. L. Bourne and J. King to American Legislative Exchange Council, Environmental Health Attendees, memorandum on the Model State Emergency Health Powers Act, November 8, 2001.

133. L. O. Gostin, *Public Health Law: Power, Duty, Restraint* (Berkeley: University of California Press; New York: Milbank Memorial Fund, 2000), p. 4; quoted in E. Salinsky, "Public Health Emergency Preparedness: Fundamentals of the 'System,'" National Health Policy Forum Background Paper, George Washington University, Washington, D.C., 2003, p. 12.

134. Moulton interview.

135. Barry Steinhardt and Andrew Schlafly, quoted in M. Hall, "Many States Reject Bioterrorism Law; Opponents Say It's Too Invasive," *USA Today*, July 23, 2002, A1.

136. G. Annas, "Bioterrorism, Public Health and Civil Liberties," *New England Journal of Medicine* 346 (2002): 1339.

137. "Public Health Surveillance," moderated by D. O'Brien, in "Public Health Legal Preparedness Workshop Summary," edited by A. Moulton and J. Hodge, January 13, 2003, www.publichealthlaw.net/Resources/ResourcesPDFs/Dec11summ.pdf, p. 2 (accessed December 10, 2005).

138. Harnish interview.

139. C. Wolfe, "Discarded Computer Had Confidential Medical Information," Associated Press State and Local Wire, February 7, 2003; see also "Kentucky Computer Awaiting Sale Held AIDS Files," *Memphis Commercial Appeal*, February 7, 2003, A7; "Kentucky: Computer Kept Files on Sexual Diseases," *New York Times*, February 7, 2003, A17; Kentucky Department of Health, "State Bioterrorism Preparedness Capacity: Key Accomplishments."

140. Interviews with Neufeld, Smith and Vossler, Rydell, Schedler, DiFerdinando, and Perrotta.

141. Chapin, "Reflections on Public Health and the War on Terrorism."

142. For further discussion of this division between federal, state, and local authorities, see Gostin, *Public Health Law*.

143. Washington [State] Emergency Management Division, "Emergency Management Assistance Compact," http://emd.wa.gov/1-dir/emac/emac-idx.htm (accessed December 15, 2005).

144. John Colmers, interview by Gerald Markowitz and David Rosner, June 27, 2003.

145. "Health Department Reports Progress on Emergency Preparedness."

146. Interviews with Schedler, Cates, Gyle, and Harnish.

147. Ohio Department of Health, "Facts about Public Health Disaster Plans" (2003).

148. Trust for America's Health, "Study Finds Federal Bioterrorism Funds Have Yielded Only Modest Improvements in States," press release, December 11, 2003, http://healthyamericans.org/newsroom/releases/release121103.pdf (accessed January 8, 2005).

149. Shelley Hearne, DrPH, Executive Director, Trust for America's Health, "Towards a National Biodefense Strategy," written testimony before the United States House of Representatives Select Committee on Homeland Security, 108th Cong., 2nd sess., June 3, 2004 (available at http://healthyamericans.org/policy/testimony/Hearne060304.pdf; accessed December 15, 2005).

150. Trust for America's Health, *Ready or Not? Protecting the Public's Health*

in the Age of Bioterrorism, 2004: Executive Summary, http://healthyamericans .org/reports/bioterror04/BioTerror04ExecSum.pdf (accessed January 8, 2006).

151. Boulton et al., "Brief Report."

152. For more on evaluation of public health preparedness, see a number of studies by the Rand Corporation, including Nicole Lurie et al., *Public Health Preparedness in California: Lessons Learned from Seven Health Jurisdictions,* electronic resource, TR-181 (Santa Monica, Calif.: RAND Corporation, 2004).

3. EMERGENCY PREPAREDNESS AND THE CDC

1. Richard Jackson, interview by David Rosner and Gerald Markowitz, May 17, 2002; all subsequent quotations from Jackson are from this interview. Information on tasks done by the CDC is from Stephen Ostroff, telephone interview by David Rosner and Gerald Markowitz, July 27, 2004; subsequent quotations from Ostroff are from this interview.

2. Jeffrey Koplan, telephone interview by Gerald Markowitz and David Rosner, June 30, 2004. All subsequent quotations from Koplan are from this interview.

3. H. C. Lane and A. S. Fauci, "Bioterrorism on the Homefront: A New Challenge for American Medicine," *Journal of the American Medical Association* 286 (2001): 2595–96; see also N. Shute et al., "Into the Zone of the Unknown," *U.S. News and World Report,* November 5, 2001, p. 40.

4. James M. Hughes to Kate Frank, e-mail, "Re: Manuscript Review," May 17, 2005.

5. James Hughes, telephone interview by Gerald Markowitz and David Rosner, October 12, 2004; all subsequent quotations from Hughes are from this interview.

The NCID was formed in the early 1980s as an amalgamation of the Bureaus of Epidemiology, Laboratories, and Tropical Diseases. Part of the rationale for the merger was to increase cooperation between epidemiologists and laboratory scientists by putting them in the same center. Anthrax and BT have reinforced the importance of this relationship between fieldwork and lab work. The NCID's mission is to prevent and control diseases and deaths caused by infectious agents, but two other groups in the CDC work on similar issues: the National Immunizations program, which deals with preventable childhood diseases, and the National Center for HIV, STD, and TB Prevention.

6. Ed Thompson, telephone interview by David Rosner and Gerald Markowitz, July 7, 2004. All subsequent quotations from Thompson are from this interview.

7. Joseph Henderson, telephone interview by David Rosner and Gerald Markowitz, June 29, 2004. All subsequent quotations from Henderson are from this interview.

8. J. L. Mothershead, K. Tonat, et al., "Bioterrorism Preparedness 3: State and Federal Programs and Response," *Emergency Medical Clinics of North America* 20 (2002): 477–500.

9. Ibid., pp. 481, 482.

10. Ibid., pp. 481–91.

11. Ibid.

12. Scott Lillibridge, telephone interview by David Rosner and Gerald Markowitz, October 5, 2004. Unless otherwise specified, all subsequent quotations from Lillibridge are from this interview.

13. S. J. J. Freedberg and M. W. Serafini, "Be Afraid, Be Moderately Afraid," *National Journal* 31 (1999): 808.

14. R. Preston, "Updating the Smallpox Vaccine," *New Yorker,* January 17, 2000, p. 27.

15. T. V. Inglesby, R. Grossman, et al., "A Plague on Your City: Observations from TOPOFF," *Clinical and Infectious Diseases* 32 (2001): 436–45.

16. A. E. Smithson and L. A. Levy, *Ataxia: The Chemical and Biological Terrorism Threat and the US Response* (Washington, D.C.: Henry L. Stimson Center, 2000); available at www.stimson.org/pub.cfm?id=12 (accessed December 10, 2005).

17. National Conference of State Legislatures, *Health Acts 2000: Summary, the Public Health Improvement Act* (2001).

18. C. W. Erickson and Bethany Barratt, "Prudence or Panic? Preparedness Exercises, Counterterror Mobilization, and Media Coverage — Dark Winter TOPOFF 1 and 2," *Journal of Homeland Security and Emergency Management* 1, no. 4 (2004): 5.

19. Scott Lillibridge, testimony before the Subcommittee on Oversight and Investigations, House Committee on Energy and Commerce, "HHS Bioterrorism Preparedness," October 10, 2001, www.hhs.gov/asp/testify/t011010a.html.

20. T. G. Thompson, "Bioterrorism: We Are Prepared, But We Can Do Better," *Vital Speeches of the Day* 68, no. 1 (2001): 6–8.

21. C. Connolly, "Smallpox Vaccine Plan Called Lacking: CDC Head Says $600 Million More Is Needed," *Washington Post,* November 30, 2001, A39.

22. Gene Matthews, telephone interview by Gerald Markowitz and David Rosner, July 6, 2004. All subsequent quotations from Matthews are from this interview.

23. "Who Will Build Our Biodefences?" *The Economist,* January 30, 2003, available at www.economist.com/displaystory.cfm?story_id=1560369 (accessed January 9, 2005).

24. George Hardy, telephone interview with David Rosner and Gerald Markowitz, August 2, 2004. All subsequent quotations from Hardy are from this interview.

25. S. Gorman and M. W. Serafini, "Homeland Security's Reality TV Show," *National Journal* 35 (2003): 1482–83.

26. Amy Smithson, quoted in M. Drexler, "The Germ Front: Experts Differ Over Whether Chemical and Biological Warfare Pose a Mass Threat — But They Agree That We Need a Stronger Public-Health Response," *American Prospect,* November 5, 2001, p. 26.

27. ASTHO, "ASTHO Survey Results on the Fiscal Status of State Public Health Preparedness Funds and the Status of State Smallpox Vaccination Program Efforts," October 27, 2003, www.astho.org/pubs/SurveyCoverNote.pdf, p. 1 (accessed January 10, 2006).

28. Trust for America's Health, *Ready or Not? Protecting the Public's Health in the Age of Bioterrorism, 2004:* Executive Summary, http://healthyamericans .org/reports/bioterror04/BioTerror04ExecSum.pdf (accessed January 8, 2006).

29. U.S. General Accounting Office, *HHS Bioterrorism Preparedness Programs: States Reported Progress but Fell Short of Program Goals for 2002,* Briefing for Congressional Staff, GAO-04–360R (Washington, D.C.: U.S. General Accounting Office, 2004), p. 24; available at www.gao.gov/new.items/d04360r .pdf (accessed December 16, 2005).

CONCLUSION

1. Joseph Henderson, telephone interview by David Rosner and Gerald Markowitz, June 29, 2004. All subsequent quotes from Henderson are from this interview.

2. Dennis Perrotta to Kate Frank, e-mail, "Review of Milbank Fund Document," October 17, 2003.

3. Michael Caldwell, "Comment on Draft," October 27, 2003.

4. M. L. Boulton, J. Abellera, J. Lemmings, and L. Robinson, "Brief Report: Terrorism and Emergency Preparedness in State and Territorial Public Health Department — United States, 2004," *Morbidity Mortality Weekly Reports* 54 (2005): 460; U.S. General Accounting Office, "HHS Bioterrorism Preparedness Programs: States Reported Progress but Fell Short of Program Goals for 2002," GAO-04–360R, February 10, 2004, www.gao.gov/new.items/d04360r.pdf (accessed January 9, 2006).

INDEX

Aaron, Barbara, 23–24, 43–44, 46
Abramovitz, Mimi, 39–40, 52
ACLU (American Civil Liberties Union),
and Model Act, 109, 112–13
AIDS, 5, 59; bioterrorism funding and,
82; budget deficits and, 89; civil
rights issues, 108, 111–12, 113–14;
federal involvement, 129; New York
City Department of Health and, 15–
16; smallpox vaccination campaign
and, 93, 100
"Air Pollution (and Deception) at Ground
Zero" (Sierra Club), 32
airport security, 88
air quality safety: everyday, 92; 9/11, 9,
13–15, 20–31, 51, 121. *See also*
chemical hazards; toxins
Akhtar, Mohammed, 56
Allen, Tom, 84
American Public Health Association
(APHA), 56, 66, 81, 102
American Red Cross, 35–36, 37, 128
Annas, George, 109
ANSER (Analytic Services) Institute for
Homeland Security, 64–65, 136
anthrax, xii, 5; cutaneous, 123; EMAC
and, 116; inhalation, 123; mock
attacks (2000), 64
anthrax episodes, 6, 16–19, 67, 100, 123;
CDC and, 17, 18, 120, 123–28, 143,
145, 146; Cipro antibiotic, 16, 17,
135; communications, 18, 58, 106,

124–28, 158, 162; Florida, 123,
143, 144, 152; labs, 78, 125, 126,
145; NBC News, 16–17, 123, 125;
New Jersey postal workers, 17,
76–77, 123, 124; New York City
Department of Health and, 16–19,
50–51; and regional coordination,
114; state public health effects, 59,
61–63, 68, 70–78, 101–2, 106,
144–45; Washington D.C. mail,
123, 124
antibiotics, 59–60; for anthrax, 16, 17,
135
Arizona: bioterrorism priority, 62, 73;
budget deficit, 84; hantavirus
pulmonary syndrome on Navaho
reservation (1993), 129, 144; and
Model Act, 111, 112; smallpox vaccination campaign, 92–93, 94, 97
Arkansas: budget deficits, 85; EMAC,
ix–x
art therapy, for traumatized children, 47
asbestos, 21, 22, 27, 28–31
Asian American Federation, 36
Associated Press, 78
Association of American Physicians and
Surgeons, 109
Association of State and Territorial
Health Officials (ASTHO), 66, 96,
106, 130, 149
Atlanta: CDC headquarters, 2, 123, 125,
126–27; mock attack, 136

Text: 10/13 Sabon
Display: Franklin Gothic
Compositor: BookMatters, Berkeley
Indexer: Barbara Roos
Printer and binder: Thomson-Shore, Inc.